DIALECTICAL BEHAVIOR THERAPY
FOR BINGE EATING AND BULIMIA

Dialectical Behavior Therapy for Binge Eating and Bulimia

DEBRA L. SAFER

CHRISTY F. TELCH

EUNICE Y. CHEN

Foreword by
Marsha M. Linehan

THE GUILFORD PRESS
New York   London

Library of Congress Cataloging-in-Publication Data

Safer, Debra L.
  Dialectical behavior therapy for binge eating and bulimia / Debra L. Safer, Christy F. Telch,
and Eunice Y. Chen.
    p. ; cm.
  Includes bibliographical references and index.
  ISBN 978-1-60623-265-1 (hardcover: alk. paper)
  ISBN 978-1-4625-3037-3 (paperback: alk. paper)
  1. Compulsive eating. 2. Bulimia. 3. Dialectical behavior therapy. I. Telch, Christy
F. II. Chen, Eunice Y. III. Title.
  [DNLM: 1. Bulimia—therapy. 2. Bulimia Nervosa—therapy. 3. Behavior Therapy—
methods. WM 175 S128d 2009]
  RC552.C65S24 2009
  616.85′26—dc22

                                                                                2009006668

About the Authors

Debra L. Safer, MD, is Assistant Professor in the Department of Psychiatry and Behavioral Sciences at Stanford University Medical Center. Dr. Safer obtained her undergraduate and master's degrees from the University of California, Berkeley. She attended medical school at the University of California, San Francisco, followed by a residency in psychiatry at Stanford University. Her postdoctoral fellowship was also at Stanford, where she worked closely with W. Stewart Agras, MD, and his eating disorders research team. Dr. Safer's research and clinical work focus on treating eating disorders in adults and adolescents utilizing dialectical behavior therapy and other empirically validated treatments.

Christy F. Telch, PhD, is in private practice in Palo Alto, California, where she focuses on treating eating disorders as well as panic and anxiety disorders. Dr. Telch obtained her undergraduate and master's degrees in psychology from California State University, Fullerton, and her PhD in counseling psychology from Stanford University. She joined the faculty of the Department of Psychiatry and Behavioral Sciences at Stanford, where she established a national reputation for her research on eating disorders, authoring or coauthoring more than 30 journal articles. In 1997, Dr. Telch received a grant from the National Institute of Mental Health for the purpose of adapting dialectical behavior therapy for the treatment of binge-eating disorder. The research she initiated with this grant and the treatment manual she wrote, *Emotion Regulation Skills Training Treatment for Binge Eating Disorder*, are the basis for this book.

Eunice Y. Chen, PhD, is Assistant Professor in the Department of Psychiatry and Behavioral Neurosciences at the University of Chicago, where she runs a dialectical behavior therapy program for adults with eating disorders. Dr. Chen received her undergraduate degree and PhD in clinical psychology from the University of Sydney, Australia. She subsequently completed postdoctoral fellowships at Yale University and at the University of Washington, with Marsha M. Linehan, PhD.

Foreword

Since the original manual for dialectical behavior therapy (DBT) was published in 1993, there has been widespread talk about adapting the treatment for different populations. I have urged researchers and clinicians to take care in how they adapt DBT, specifically, that they not reach beyond the data, that they stay as close to the manual as possible, and that they conduct research on their adaptations. Many people have been trying to adapt DBT for different populations, but very few have done so with the diligence of Debra Safer, Christy Telch, and Eunice Chen. *Dialectical Behavior Therapy for Binge Eating and Bulimia* is, to date, the only DBT treatment manual for eating disorders that has data from randomized controlled trials to support it.

Christy Telch approached me in 1994 about adapting DBT for binge-eating disorder. She first wanted to ensure that she was competent in standard DBT before adapting the treatment, so she began supervision with me. Christy is one of those rare people who understands DBT from the inside out. She not only has a grasp of the strategies and principles of DBT, she also understands its nuances and has incorporated them into this book.

Debra Safer, an important member of a committee for strategic planning of DBT research that I formed several years ago, soon became involved in developing the book. Debra understands both eating disorders and DBT and has a passion for ensuring that this book stays true to the data and the treatment.

Eunice Chen joined the Behavioral Research and Therapy Clinics (BRTC) at the University of Washington in 2002 as a postdoctoral fellow. She has become an expert in eating disorders, especially as they are part of complex, multiple-problem patients. While at the BRTC, Eunice studied DBT and eating disorders as well as borderline personality disorder (BPD). She has since left the BRTC and moved to the University of Chicago, where she is doing exciting research with various eating disorders, BPD, and DBT.

Every week, we field phone calls and e-mails from people who are looking for innovative ways to treat eating disorders. Most clinicians and researchers have believed that DBT could be adapted for eating disorders, especially when the disordered eating behaviors were the consequence of emotion dysregulation. Safer, Telch, and Chen are the first to do so with an empirical basis. Prior to the release of this book, many clinicians have been using the standard skills training handouts with people with bulimia and binge eating. This book provides over 30 handouts that remain true to the original DBT skills, but are written to address eating behaviors. The case examples are tailored to bingeing and bulimic behaviors and will guide clinicians and researchers in providing DBT.

As you read this book, there are several important things to consider. First, this is not the treatment manual for complex, suicidal patients. The data for suicidal patients still support standard DBT. Second, this book is for stage 3, single-problem patients. It is skills training group based and is tailored for patients with bulimia and binge eating. Third, this book does not currently have data for treating anorexia. As always, it is important to follow the data.

Best wishes in your efforts to provide and research DBT.

MARSHA M. LINEHAN, PhD
Professor, Department of Psychology
Director, Behavioral Research and Therapy Clinics
University of Washington

Acknowledgments

We are deeply grateful to the many individuals who have helped to make this book a reality, including those serving as therapists on our research trials: Brenda Brownlow, PhD, Emily Hugo, PsyD, Rebecca Klein, PsyD, and Susan Wiser, PhD; those serving as research assistants over the years: Wanda Chui, Sara Clancy, Molly McMillen, Shireen Rizvi, PhD, and Amanda Vaught; and the many doctoral students who assisted with the project, among them Maggie Chartier, MPH, Megan Jones, Megan McElheran, and Nicole Riddle. Others who made significant contributions are W. Stewart Agras, MD, Jennifer Couturier, MD, Kara Fitzpatrick, PhD, Craig Forte, LCSW, Eval Gal-Oz, PhD, Gerry Gelbart, MD, James Gross, PhD, James Lock, MD, PhD, and Lynda Malavanya, MD.

We also wish to thank Shari Manning, PhD, of Behavioral Tech Research, Inc., for her generosity in both reading the manuscript and offering valuable feedback. We acknowledge, with gratitude, our debt to Marsha M. Linehan, PhD, whose own work inspired this adaptation and whose encouragement motivated us to publish. And we have been immensely fortunate to have Kitty Moore as our editor at The Guilford Press; her expert guidance is felt throughout this book.

Debra L. Safer would also like to thank her loving family, with special gratitude to Dan and Elaine, her parents; her husband Adam and their daughter, Zoe; and Vilma, their indispensable nanny.

Christy F. Telch would like to personally thank Drs. W. Stewart Agras, Bruce Arnow, and Marsha M. Linehan for their encouragement, support, and wise counsel throughout the process of conducting this work. Additionally, she would like to express her heartfelt appreciation to her loving husband, Bob Forman, and dear sons, Aaron Telch and James Forman, for their generosity of spirit and unending patience throughout her work on this project and her career.

Eunice Y. Chen would like to thank Mike McCloskey and Sunny Koey for their love and support.

Finally, all of us want to specially acknowledge and thank all the clients who participated in our research trials over the years. Without you, this book would never have been possible.

Contents

Introduction   1

CHAPTER 1.   Binge-Eating Disorder and Bulimia Nervosa: 5
Why Dialectical Behavior Therapy?

CHAPTER 2.   Orientation for Therapists   16

CHAPTER 3.   The Pretreatment Stage: The Pretreatment Interview   30
and Introductory Sessions

CHAPTER 4.   Mindfulness Core Skills   89

CHAPTER 5.   Emotion Regulation Skills   120

CHAPTER 6.   Distress Tolerance Skills   155

CHAPTER 7.   Final Sessions: Review and Relapse Prevention   179

CHAPTER 8.   Illustrative Case Examples   190

CHAPTER 9.   Future Directions   215

APPENDIX.   Information for Researchers   223

References   229

Index   237

Purchasers of this book can download and print select
appendices at *www.guilford.com/safer-forms* for personal use or
use with individual clients (see copyright page for details).

Introduction

This book was written in response to repeated requests from therapists in the clinical and research community for a detailed description of how dialectical behavior therapy (DBT) has been adapted to treat binge-eating disorder (BED) and symptoms of bulimia nervosa (BN). The aim of this book is to make available a comprehensive presentation of this promising treatment.

The treatment program is based on the original manual written by Christy F. Telch (1997a). This program has been tested and shown to be efficacious in a number of research studies conducted at the Department of Psychiatry and Behavioral Sciences at Stanford University (Safer, Robinson, & Jo, in press; Safer, Telch, & Agras, 2001a, 2001b; Telch, 1997b; Telch, Agras, & Linehan, 2000, 2001).

The program described in this book is an adaptation of standard DBT, a treatment originally developed by Linehan (1993a, 1993b) for individuals engaging in recurrent suicidal behavior who meet criteria for borderline personality disorder. This adapted version for eating disorders involves a number of modifications to standard DBT that reflect the differing client populations and research questions. For instance, standard DBT was developed to address the severity and potential lethality of behaviors commonly associated with borderline personality. A year-long treatment, standard DBT includes weekly individual psychotherapy, weekly group skills training, access to 24-hour telephone coaching, and a weekly consultation team for therapists.

Our adapted version of DBT is aimed at clients whose BED or BN symptoms are the primary focus of treatment. This adapted version combines elements of the functions of two distinct modalities in standard DBT: individual psychotherapy (enhancement of motivation) and group skills training (acquisition/strengthening of new skills). These are delivered in 20 weekly sessions, a 2-hour group format for clients with BED or a 1-hour individual format for clients with BN symptoms. In addition, this adapted version of DBT includes three of the four skills training modules of standard program DBT (Mindfulness, Emotion Regulation, Distress

1

Tolerance). The rationale for excluding the Interpersonal Effectiveness skills module was based on clinical trial design concerns regarding potential overlap with other treatments developed for BED and BN that specifically focus upon treating interpersonal problems.

FOR WHOM IS THIS BOOK WRITTEN?

We have written this book for a variety of different audiences. For therapists with training in DBT but little experience with treating disordered eating, this book is intended to provide pertinent eating-disorder background, as well as specific direction for applying DBT with clients whose primary presenting symptoms are binge eating or bulimia. For therapists familiar with treating clients with eating disorders but not with DBT, this book outlines the basic principles of DBT with a focus on how these are adapted for individuals with binge-eating and purging problems. For investigators interested in researching DBT as adapted for BED and BN, we hope that the detailed description of this treatment modification will increase its use, encourage program improvements, and further treatment evaluation efforts.

One important note of caution. By documenting DBT adapted for BED and BN, we do not wish to convey an oversimplification of the treatment or the problems it is intended to address. The issues our clients face are complicated, and DBT is a multifaceted treatment approach. In order to ensure competent delivery of this treatment, we recommend a sound background in general cognitive-behavioral principles and an understanding of standard DBT. We consider Linehan's two manuals, *Cognitive-Behavioral Treatment of Borderline Personality Disorder* (Linehan, 1993a) and *Skills Training Manual for Treating Borderline Personality Disorder* (Linehan, 1993b), to be companion texts to this book and recommend that they be read prior to embarking on this treatment.

WHAT TYPES OF CLIENTS MIGHT MOST BENEFIT FROM RECEIVING THIS TREATMENT?

This treatment was originally developed and studied in an outpatient setting in which clients with BED received weekly group sessions and clients with bingeing and purging symptoms received weekly individual sessions. Applying the treatment in similar settings with similar clients would have the greatest likelihood of reproducing the positive outcomes originally found. Clinicians and researchers interested in using or evaluating this treatment in other contexts, such as a partial hospital or inpatient ward setting, will probably need to make further modifications.

The research support for DBT adapted for BED and BN, although promising, is relatively limited. Thus, we advise proceeding with the use of this treatment after carefully considering the available alternatives. The most conservative recommendation at this time is that DBT as adapted for binge eating and bulimic behavior may be most appropriate for clients who have undergone the standard, evidence-based eating-disorder treatments (e.g., cognitive-behavioral therapy or interpersonal psychotherapy) and failed to improve or received minimal benefit.

To date, research has not identified the relevant variables for matching clients and DBT adapted for eating disorders in order to produce the best outcomes. Therefore, until such research is conducted, we can only speculate about the factors that might suggest a good match between the treatment described in this book and a particular client. For instance, the treatment model underlying this adapted DBT approach posits a primary link between affect dysregulation and binge-eating or bulimic behaviors. For a client struggling with emotional eating who describes binge-eating episodes clearly triggered by negative emotions (e.g., anger, sadness), this treatment may be particularly suitable. Anecdotally, we have found that clients who report that the Emotion Regulation model of binge eating fits their own personal experience seem to do particularly well.

CLIENTS WE RECOMMEND NOT RECEIVE THIS ADAPTED DBT TREATMENT

It is not unusual for clients seeking treatment for BED or BN to suffer from comorbid conditions such as mood disorders (e.g., Berkman, Lohr, & Bulik, 2007; Telch & Stice, 1998) and Axis II disorders (e.g., Cassin & von Ranson, 2005). Data from our own treatment studies demonstrate significant improvement in target symptoms in clients despite substantial comorbidity rates for depression, anxiety, substance abuse, and personality disorders (see Table I.1). With clients with multiple symptoms, it is always advisable to prioritize treatment targets. Accordingly, if other serious behaviors, such as current substance abuse or dependence or suicidal behaviors, are present, we recommend postponing the use of DBT for BED or BN treatment until the eating-disorder symptoms are the appropriate primary treatment target (Chen, Matthews, Allen, Kuo, & Linehan, 2008). That is to say, we would not recommend this adapted DBT approach for clients with severely chronic multiple symptoms who are also actively suicidal or who have borderline personality disorder or combined borderline personality disorder with substance dependence. For these individuals, the standard DBT program has a number of randomized clinical trials (Linehan, Armstrong, Suarez, Allmon, & Heard, 1991; Linehan et al., 1999; Turner, 2000; Koons et al., 2001; Linehan, Dimeff, et al., 2002; Verheul et al., 2003; Linehan et al., 2006) and a number of nonrandomized controlled trials (Barley et al., 1993; Bohus et al., 2000; Stanley, Ivanoff, Brodsky, Oppenheim, & Mann, 1998; McCann, Ball, & Ivanoff, 2000; Rathus & Miller, 2002;

TABLE I.1. Rates of Comorbid Psychopathology among Clients in Randomized DBT for BED Study

Comorbid condition	Percentage (%)
Major depression (current)	9
Major depression (lifetime)	38
Anxiety disorder (current)	18
Anxiety disorder (lifetime)	35
Substance abuse/dependence (lifetime)	27
Personality disorder	27

Note. Data from Telch, Agras, and Linehan (2001).

Bohus, Haaf, & Simms, 2004) attesting to its efficacy. The original comprehensive multimodal DBT program would be the treatment of choice for such clients. Similarly, individuals with active substance abuse or dependence may be best directed to a specific substance abuse or dependence treatment.

There are also currently no published empirical data examining the efficacy of this program for clients meeting criteria for anorexia nervosa, although there are programs adapting DBT for these individuals (Wisniewski, Safer, & Chen, 2007).

ORGANIZATION OF THIS BOOK

This book consists of nine chapters. The first chapter familiarizes readers with the many problems faced by people with BED and BN, gives an overview of currently available treatments, and provides the rationale and existing evidence for adapting DBT for BED and BN.

Chapter 2 orients therapists to DBT for BED and BN. It explains the impetus for developing this adapted treatment; includes a brief review of standard DBT's empirical evidence; introduces the treatment model, assumptions, goals, and targets; and describes basic therapist strategies and specifics regarding how sessions are structured.

Chapters 3 to 7 describe the "nuts and bolts" of how DBT was adapted to treat BED and bulimic symptoms. Chapter 3 focuses on the pretreatment and introductory sessions. The Mindfulness module is outlined in Chapter 4, the Emotion Regulation module in Chapter 5, and the Distress Tolerance module in Chapter 6. Chapter 7 describes treatment termination and relapse prevention.

Chapter 8 uses two case examples, one of a client with BN and another of clients with BED treated in a group format, to illustrate the delivery of the treatment and common issues that arise.

Finally, Chapter 9 outlines future directions for DBT for BED and BN.

The Appendix at the end of the book offers detail on criteria used for recruiting participants for our randomized trials, the number and type of diagnostic assessments, and specifics regarding the therapeutic content (e.g., skills taught) during each of the 20 research sessions.

A WORD BEFORE WE GET STARTED

We recommend that therapists planning to deliver this treatment should do two things (in addition to reading Linehan's manuals). First, we recommend reading the entire book prior to conducting treatment with clients, paying close attention to the treatment rationale and treatment goals as described in Chapter 2. Second, before teaching the skills to others, therapists should have practice using each of the skills on their own. Therapists should continue to practice the skills when delivering the treatment and engage in "homework" practice of the specific skills that are the focus of the session.

CHAPTER 1

Binge-Eating Disorder and Bulimia Nervosa

Why Dialectical Behavior Therapy?

This chapter explores the many problems faced by people with binge-eating disorder (BED) and bulimia nervosa (BN), focusing on key features of these disorders, as well as on their associated impairments to one's psychological, physical, and social functioning. Although treatment with current leading therapies, such as cognitive-behavioral therapy (CBT), interpersonal psychotherapy (IPT), and behavioral weight loss therapy (BWL) offers significant improvement, the fact that a sizeable number of clients remain symptomatic after these treatments has prompted the development of other therapy models. We present support for one such model, an affect regulation model of binge eating and purging. This includes outlining the rationale for adapting dialectical behavior therapy (DBT), originally developed to target affect dysregulation among individuals with borderline personality disorder, to treat disordered eating behaviors. We conclude with a summary of the available research evidence for the efficacy of DBT for BED and BN.

OVERVIEW

BED and BN, the two eating disorders for which the treatment described in this book has been researched in randomized trials, are both typified by binge eating. Two components determine whether an eating episode is a binge: the quantity of food eaten and the presence of an accompanying sense of lack of control (American Psychiatric Association, 2000). In other words, the amount of food consumed over a discrete time period (e.g., 2 hours) should be unusually large compared with what most people would eat in the same time period under similar circumstances. In addition, during the episode, a lack of control is felt, as if one could not stop eating or control what or how much is eaten. BN is distinguished from BED by the use

5

of compensatory behaviors (e.g., vomiting, extreme dietary restriction, laxative or diuretic misuse, overexercise) in response to binge eating.

BINGE-EATING DISORDER

BED is currently listed in the appendix of the text revision of the fourth edition of the *Diagnostic and Statistical Manual of Mental Disorders* (DSM-IV-TR; American Psychiatric Association, 2000) as a research diagnosis requiring further study. The proposed criteria for the diagnosis include the occurrence of binge eating approximately 2 days per week for a minimum period of 6 months in the absence of compensatory behaviors. Other associated features include eating much more quickly than normal, eating to the point of physical discomfort, eating despite lack of physical hunger, eating alone due to embarrassment about one's amount of food intake, and feeling disgust, depression, or guilt after binge eating.

About 2–5% of the general population suffers from BED (Bruce & Agras, 1992; Fairburn, Cooper, Doll, Norman, & O'Connor, 2000; Spitzer et al., 1992, 1993). Its prevalence is even higher among certain groups of individuals, such as those seeking treatment for weight control (20–40%; Spitzer et al., 1992, 1993; Brody, Walsh, & Devlin, 1994). Of those undergoing bariatric surgery, up to 49% meet criteria for BED (see reviews by de Zwaan et al., 2003; Niego, Kofman, Weiss, & Geliebter, 2007). And among members of Overeaters Anonymous, rates of those suffering from BED have been estimated to reach 71% (Spitzer et al., 1992).

BED is more common in women. However, a notable number of men also suffer with this disorder. The ratio of males to females is 2:3 among overweight individuals with BED and approaches 1:1 in community samples (Spitzer et al., 1992).

People diagnosed with BED typically describe a lifetime struggle with both their binge-eating symptoms and issues of weight control. By midadolescence or early adulthood, the onset of binge eating, dieting, and overweight has usually occurred (Spurrell, Wilfley, Tanofsky, & Brownell, 1997), and, unfortunately, these often become ongoing concerns. In one large study of individuals with BED, three-quarters reported having spent more than half their adult lives on diets, and about half had gained and lost at least 20 pounds five times or more (Spitzer et al., 1993).

Although some individuals with BED have normal weight, people meeting criteria for BED are more likely to be overweight or obese (e.g., Bruce & Agras, 1992). Indeed, a number of studies (Bruce & Agras, 1992; Spitzer et al., 1993; Telch, Agras, & Rossiter, 1988) have shown a positive association between the frequency of binge eating and the degree of obesity as measured by body mass index (BMI; kg/m^2). Despite this overlap between binge eating and obesity, important differences exist between people with BED and weight-matched individuals (i.e., those who are equally overweight) who do not meet BED criteria. These differences span multiple domains, including psychiatric and eating-disorder-specific disturbances, social and work-related impairments, and physical consequences—as discussed in the following sections.

Adding to the serious difficulties faced by clients with BED, carrying the diagnosis of BED predicts a worsened outcome in response to weight loss treatment. For example, overweight participants with BED enrolled in a weight loss clinic attained only 55% of the weight loss achieved by their fellow participants without BED (Pagoto et al., 2007). A review by Niego and colleagues (2007) of bariatric surgery patients showed that those with significant binge-eating histories were more likely to have a poorer outcome—including greater likelihood of suffering from disordered eating after surgery (Hsu, Betancourt, & Sullivan, 1996; Hsu, Sullivan, & Benotti, 1997), smaller loss of initial excess weight (Sallet et al., 2007), higher levels of weight regain (Hsu et al., 1996), and greater requirements for postoperative adjustments (Busetto et al., 2005).

Psychiatric and Eating-Disorder-Specific Symptomatology in BED

Carrying a diagnosis of BED is associated with higher levels of psychiatric symptoms compared with weight-matched controls without BED. In a study that examined non-treatment-seeking individuals, the rates of lifetime major depression (49%), as well as of any Axis I diagnosis (59%), were about twice those found in overweight/obese controls without BED (28% and 37%, respectively; Telch & Stice, 1998). Another large study found that overweight individuals with BED, as compared with overweight individuals without BED, were more likely to have a history of alcohol abuse (15% versus 1.7%) or drug abuse (13% versus 4%; Spitzer et al., 1993).

In terms of personality disorders, the likelihood of being diagnosed with any Axis II disorder was found to be four times higher (20%) in those with BED than in overweight/obese controls (5%; Telch & Stice, 1998). Both Cluster B (e.g., borderline personality disorder) and Cluster C (e.g., avoidant personality disorder, obsessive–compulsive personality disorder) were significantly more prevalent (Specker et al., 1994).

Of note, research has also shown that the degree of co-occurring psychological disorders is related to binge-eating severity rather than to degree of overweight (Picot & Lilenfeld, 2003; Telch & Agras, 1994; Yanovski, Nelson, Dubbert, & Spitzer, 1993). Indeed, rates of co-occurring psychiatric disorders among obese individuals without BED are similar to rates in a nonpatient community sample (Spitzer et al., 1993; Telch & Stice, 1998).

In addition to increased rates of psychiatric symptoms, those with BED also demonstrate higher levels of eating-disorder-specific pathology. For example, individuals with BED report greater overconcern about weight and shape (Eldredge & Agras, 1996; Spitzer et al., 1993), more fears of weight gain, a higher preoccupation with food and weight, and greater body dissatisfaction (e.g., Wilson, Nonas, & Rosenblum, 1993). Importantly, these eating-disorder-specific symptoms, such as overconcern with weight and shape, have been shown to be independent of actual body weight (e.g., Eldredge & Agras, 1996).

Social and Occupational Impairment in BED

People with BED are also more likely to show impaired social and occupational functioning. Spitzer and colleagues (Spitzer et al., 1993) found that 65.1% of participants with BED, compared with 28.8% of weight-matched controls, reported impaired interpersonal relationships due to distress about their eating and weight. Similarly, reports of work impairment due to eating and weight-related distress were more than double in those with BED (44.5%) compared with weight-matched individuals without the disorder (17.3%; Spitzer et al., 1993).

Other investigators examining the impact of BED on quality of life found significantly higher ratings of overall distress among obese individuals with BED compared with obese individuals without the disorder (Rieger, Wilfley, Stein, Marino, & Crow, 2005). When asked to assess the effects of being overweight on specific domains of quality of life, those with BED reported significantly more impairment in the psychosocial domains of work (e.g., receiving appropriate raises), public activities (e.g., worrying about fitting into seats in public spaces), sexual life (e.g., sexual desire), and self-esteem (Rieger et al., 2005). Because the participants with and without BED were comparable in terms of degree of overweight, these findings could not be attributed to elevated levels of obesity (Rieger et al., 2005).

Physiological Consequences of BED

As noted, people with BED are more likely to be overweight or obese than individuals without BED. Also, the greater the severity of binge eating—in terms of its frequency and size—the higher the degree of overweight, as measured by the BMI (Bruce & Agras, 1992; Picot & Lilenfeld, 2003; Telch et al., 1988). (Normal is defined as a BMI between 18.5 and 24.9, overweight as a BMI between 25 and 29.9, and obesity as a BMI of 30 or greater [National Heart, Lung, and Blood Institute and the National Institutes of Health, 1998].) In a community sample of 455 women, for example, women who met full criteria for BED had higher average body weights (BMI = 30.24) than those who binged less than two times per week (BMI = 26.21), and the BMIs of this latter group were higher than among those who did not binge at all (BMI = 22.85; Bruce & Agras, 1992).

Not surprisingly given the overlap between BED and obesity, individuals with this disorder are more likely to suffer from the significant medical problems associated with obesity itself (e.g., hypertension, stroke, heart disease, sleep apnea, colon cancer, breast cancer; National Heart, Lung, and Blood Institute, 1998; Pi-Sunyer, 2002). This association highlights the prominent public health implications of BED. In some instances, the presence of binge eating appears to confer additional medical consequences above and beyond those accounted for by obesity alone. For example, rates of Type II diabetes were 14% among those binge eating at least two times per week compared with 4% in controls matched for BMI and age (Kenardy, Mensch, Bowen, & Pearson, 1994). In addition, a significant relationship was found between glycemic control (as measured by HbA1$_c$) and binge eating among Type II diabetics with BED—a relationship that was independent of weight (Kenardy, Mensch, Bowen, & Dalton, 2001). Further evidence of the serious physical consequences associated with a diagnosis of BED is the overall health status of participants with BED, which is significantly lower than U.S. norms and even lower than that of obese weight-matched controls (Hsu et al., 2002).

Emotions, Affect Regulation, and BED

Research evidence highlights the role emotions (particularly negative emotions) and affect regulation play in binge eating. For example, the most frequently cited precipitants of binge eating are stress and negative mood (Polivy & Herman, 1993). Furthermore, overweight binge eaters report higher urges to binge in response to negative emotions than those who do not binge eat, irrespective of level of over-weight (Eldredge & Agras, 1996). In a study examining which of six emotions are most associated with triggering binge eating, anxiety was the most frequently cited, followed by sadness, loneliness, tiredness, anger, and happiness (Masheb & Grilo, 2006).

In an experimental study of women with BED and weight-matched controls, negative emotional states were associated with both loss of control and an eating episode labeled as a binge (Telch & Agras, 1996). And an experimental study that manipulated caloric deprivation and the conditions for inducing a negative or a neutral mood noted the self-defined binges of obese women with BED to be signifi-cantly associated with negative mood rather than with caloric deprivation (Agras & Telch, 1998). Other experiments describe similar findings regarding the role of negative mood in triggering binge eating (Chua, Touyz, & Hill, 2004).

A study that utilized experience sampling from participants who tracked their moods and eating behaviors with handheld computers over 6 days reported that more aversive moods preceded binge eating in participants with BED compared with weight-matched controls without BED (Greeno, Wing, & Shiffman, 2000). Furthermore, at random prompts throughout the course of the study, participants with BED indicated experiencing a significantly worse mood on average than par-ticipants without BED. Greater diurnal fluctuations in depression and anxiety were recorded among binge eaters assessed during a 2-week period (Lingswiler, Crowther, & Stephens, 1987). The binge eaters, whether of normal weight or over-weight, also described negative moods as more frequent during eating and binge-eating episodes than did non-binge-eating participants (Lingswiler et al., 1987). In addition to being more likely to eat in response to negative moods, there is evidence that binge eaters evaluate situations as being more stressful than do non-binge eaters (Hansel & Wittrock, 1997).

A potential reason that binge eaters eat in response to negative moods and judge situations as more stressful may be that they have deficits in the ability to regulate their emotions. Supporting evidence for the role of emotion dysregulation in binge eaters was found by Whiteside and colleagues (2007), who reported that difficulties in identifying and making sense of emotional states, along with limited access to emotion regulation strategies, were associated with binge eating over and above the effects of gender, food restriction, and overevaluation of weight and shape.

BULIMIA NERVOSA

BN is marked by a preoccupation with thinness and episodes of binge eating fol-lowed by compensatory behaviors (e.g., vomiting, extreme dietary restriction, lax-ative or diuretic abuse, overexercise). To establish the diagnosis, these episodes must have occurred at least twice a week on average during the prior 3 months. The disorder is not diagnosed within the context of anorexia nervosa, and most clients are of normal weight.

The onset of BN typically occurs in adolescence or early adulthood and is often precipitated by dieting (American Psychiatric Association, 2000). Females make up the majority (90%) of those diagnosed (American Psychiatric Association, 2000), with approximately 1 in 100 women meeting criteria for BN (Hoek & van Hoeken, 2003; Hsu, 1996). Rates of BN may be higher within certain subgroups. For instance of college women in the United States, 2 to 4 in 100 may be affected (Katzman & Wolchick, 1984; Healy, Conroy, & Walsh, 1985; Pyle, Halvorson, Neuman, & Mitchell, 1986; Drewnowski, Yee, & Krahn, 1988; Pyle, Neuman, Halvorson, & Mitchell, 1991).

BN has a chronic course that is likely to be unstable (Fairburn et al., 2000), with waxing and waning periods of binge eating and purging over time (Milos, Spindler, Schnyder, & Fairburn, 2005; Wilson, Grilo, & Vitousek, 2007). Rates of remission range from an estimated 31% to 74% (Ben-Tovim et al., 2001; Grilo et al., 2003; Milos et al., 2005; Wilson et al., 2007). When remission takes place, it tends to be time-limited, so that relapse is common (Ben-Tovim et al., 2001; Herzog et al., 1999; Wilson et al., 2007).

Like BED, BN is associated with impairments in psychiatric, social, and physical functioning. These are elaborated in the following sections.

Psychiatric and Eating-Disorder-Specific Symptomatology in BN

People with BN frequently suffer from co-occurring Axis I (e.g., mood, anxiety, substance use) and Axis II (e.g., borderline personality, obsessive–compulsive) psychiatric disorders. Although estimates of prevalence vary across studies, reviews of the literature have found higher rates of lifetime depression (e.g., 60–70%) in patients with BN (Godart et al., 2007) than in the general community (16.2%; Kessler et al., 2003), particularly when larger sample sizes are studied. Comorbid anxiety in individuals with BN is also more common than in controls, with lifetime prevalence rates of least one anxiety disorder (e.g., obsessive–compulsive disorder, social phobia, posttraumatic stress disorder) ranging from 25 to 75% (Swinbourne & Touyz, 2007). Interestingly, the onset of the anxiety disorder in most cases precedes that of the BN (Swinbourne & Touyz, 2007). Co-occurring alcohol abuse or dependence is also very common, with a rate of 46% found by Bulik and colleagues (2004). Rates of lifetime substance abuse also appear elevated in women with BN, ranging from 18% (Herzog et al., 2006) to 28% (Lacey, 1993). Lifetime rates of alcohol abuse and substance use disorders in individuals with BN are higher than in the general community (13.2% and 14.6%, respectively; Kessler et al., 2005).

Rates of personality disorders, particularly Cluster B types, have also been shown to be greater in people with BN. In a review of prevalence rates derived from diagnostic interviews (a more stringent assessment method than self-report), borderline personality disorder rates were 6–37%, and avoidant personality disorder rates were 2–36% (Cassin & von Ranson, 2005). In comparison, prevalence rates in community samples have been reported at 0.5% for borderline personality disorder and 1.8% for avoidant personality disorder (Samuels et al., 2002).

As to eating-disorder-specific psychopathology, people with BN, compared with non-eating-disordered controls, report significantly higher levels of concerns regarding body shape, body weight, eating (e.g., preoccupation with food and calories), and dietary restriction (Cooper, Cooper, & Fairburn, 1989).

Social Impairment and BN

BN affects social adjustment. For instance, individuals with BN, compared with non-eating-disordered controls, depict more overall social impairment, specifically in the areas of work, leisure, and family relationships (Herzog, Keller, Lavori, & Ott, 1987). Women whose BN is active, compared with women whose BN is in remission and with non-eating-disordered controls, report significantly less emotional support (Rorty, Yager, Buckwalter, & Rossotto, 1999). And both those with active or remitted BN, compared with non-eating-disordered controls, expressed significant dissatisfaction with the quality of emotional support provided by relatives (Rorty et al., 1999). The social impairment experienced by patients with BN appears to be enduring. Ten years after being diagnosed with BN, women continued to experience difficulties in their interpersonal relationships (Keel, Mitchell, Miller, Davis, & Crow, 2000).

Studies of quality of life in BN show that individuals with a history of BN versus those without such a history report more difficulties, particularly with emotional functioning (Doll, Petersen, & Stewart-Brown, 2005). Compared with a group of individuals with mood disorders, eating-disordered patients, including patients with BN, reported having a worsened quality of life (de la Rie, Noordenbos, & van Furth, 2005). These differences in quality of life seem long-standing, with former eating-disordered patients having a poorer quality of life than a control reference group (de la Rie et al., 2005).

Physiological Consequences of BN

BN is associated with serious physiological consequences, especially among those who regularly vomit or engage in laxative abuse. Though mortality due to BN is low, it is not insignificant. Crude mortality rates due to all causes range from 0.3% to 2% (Fichter, Quadflieg, & Hedlund, 2008; Keel & Mitchell, 1997). Potentially life-threatening complications include low potassium (hypokalemia), esophageal ruptures, cathartic colon, impaired kidney function, cardiac arrythmias, and cardiac arrest (Kaplan & Garfinkel, 1993; Sansone & Sansone, 1994).

In one study of 275 women with BN, the most common complaints were weakness (84%), bloating (75%), cheek puffiness (50%), dental symptoms (36%), and finger calluses (27%; Mitchell, Hatsukami, Eckert, & Pyle, 1985). Even when not directly life threatening, bulimic behaviors profoundly affect the body in terms of oral complications, gastrointestinal symptoms, renal and electrolyte abnormalities, cardiovascular symptoms, and negative consequences to the endocrine system (see, e.g., reviews by Mehler, Crews, & Weiner, 2004; Mitchell & Crow, 2006). Erosion of teeth enamel, for example, is usually seen within 6 months of self-induced vomiting and is always evident in those suffering for 5 or more years (Althshuler, Dechow, Waller, & Hardy, 1990). Parotid gland enlargement is estimated to affect between 10 and 50% patients with BN (Mehler et al., 2004). Hypokalemia occurs in approximately 14% of bulimic patients. This serious electrolyte disturbance may potentially lead to other complications, such as cardiac arrythmias and the degeneration of cardiac muscle (Casiero & Frishman, 2006). In terms of endocrine system involvement, although evidence for a causal relationship between bulimia and diabetes is mixed, it is clear that the presence of an eating disorder in addition to diabetes is linked to a worsened diabetic course—including the development of end-organ damage at a younger age (Rydall, Rodin, Olmsted, Devenyi, & Daneman, 1997).

Emotions, Affect Regulation, and BN

Aversive emotions may bring about, maintain, and be a consequence of BN behaviors. Bulimic behaviors are frequently related to negative affective states, including anxiety, depression, and anger (e.g., Abraham & Beumont, 1982; Arnow, Kenardy, & Agras, 1995; Stice, Killen, Hayward, & Taylor, 1998). In a study recording 2 weeks of data from participants with BN who were given handheld computers, lower mood (less positive affect, more negative affect, higher anger/hostility, and higher stress) was reported on days when binge eating and vomiting occurred (Smyth et al., 2007). Within single days, the researchers noted a worsened mood trajectory over the hours prior to a binge–purge episode and a sharply improved mood trajectory following the event. These findings help explain the persistence of BN behaviors in the short run despite their not being an effective overall coping strategy. In other words, the average "best" mood on a binge–purge day was still more negative than the mood on days on which no binge–purge occurred. However, within a few hours after the event, binge and purge behaviors are strongly negatively reinforced by allowing escape or avoidance of strongly negative affective states (Smyth et al., 2007). These results are supported by other researchers (e.g., Lingswiler, Crowther, & Stephens, 1989; Lynch, Everingham, Dubitzky, Harman, & Kassert, 2000; Powell & Thelen, 1996; Steiger et al., 2005). Likewise, purging or laxative use in individuals with BN has been shown to reduce negative affect prompted by binge eating (e.g., Powell & Thelen, 1996).

Self-report studies suggest that, in addition to increased negative mood on binge–purge days, individuals with BN have higher levels of depression (Bulik, Lawson, & Carter, 1996) and anger (Waller et al., 2003) and more fluctuating moods (Johnson & Larson, 1982). Individuals with BN may also have deficits in the processing of emotions. For instance, participants with BN, compared with controls, show attentional deficits, including paying selective attention to emotionally laden words (e.g., body shape or weight and food-related words) when using the Stroop paradigm (Dobson & Dozois, 2004), the visual probe paradigm (Rieger et al., 1998), and the dichotic listening task paradigm (Schotte, McNally, & Turner, 1990). When presented food cues in experimental paradigms, participants with BN, compared with those without BN, indicate greater anxiety (Bulik et al., 1996) and have a potentiated startle reflex, suggesting strong negative affect (Mauler, Hamm, Weike, & Tuschen-Caffier, 2006). In addition, participants with BN compared with normal controls, endorse greater difficulties with self-awareness of emotions (Legenbauer, Vocks, & Ruddel, 2008). Along with other eating-disordered populations, they report more difficulties with distress tolerance than do women without histories of an eating disorder (Corstorphine, Mountford, Tomlinson, Waller, & Meyer, 2007).

For those wishing further information about eating disorders and obesity, excellent overviews are available in Fairburn and Brownell (2001) and Garner and Garfinkel (1997).

RATIONALE FOR DEVELOPMENT OF DBT AS ADAPTED FOR BED AND BN

Existing treatments can ameliorate symptoms of BED and BN. These include (1) CBT (Fairburn, 1995; Marcus, 1997; Wilson, Fairburn, & Agras, 1997), which focuses on normalizing disordered eating patterns (i.e., decreasing dietary restraint) and tackling overvalued ideas regarding weight and shape; (2) IPT (Klerman & Weissman, 1993; Wilfley et al., 1993; Wilfley et al., 2002), which aims to resolve interpersonal problems that maintain disordered eating; and (3) BWL (Agras et al., 1994; Marcus, Wing, & Fairburn, 1995; Munsch et al., 2007), which stresses decreasing the chaotic eating patterns and the overconsumption of calories characteristic of obese clients with BED. Although such treatments address emotions (e.g., an IPT focus on interpersonal role disputes or grief would address negative emotions), none directly focuses both theoretically and specifically on the role of negative emotions in BED and BN.

The fact that a significant number of clients with BED and BN continue to suffer from their eating-disorder symptoms either at posttreatment with CBT, IPT, or BWL or over the period following treatment (Wilson et al., 2007) calls for other theoretical conceptualizations and/or treatment approaches for BED and BN. One such model is the affect regulation model. Drawing on an extensive literature that links negative affect and disordered eating (Abraham & Beumont, 1982; Arnow, Kenardy, & Agras, 1992, 1995; Polivy & Herman, 1993), the affect regulation model conceptualizes binge eating and other types of eating pathology (e.g., vomiting, restrictive eating) as behavioral attempts to influence, change, or control painful emotional states (Linehan & Chen, 2005; Waller, 2003; Wiser & Telch, 1999; Wisniewski & Kelly, 2003). The binge episodes appear to function in both BED and BN by providing negative reinforcement or momentary relief from these aversive emotions (Arnow et al., 1995; Polivy & Herman, 1993; Smyth et al., 2007; Stickney, Miltenberger, & Wolff, 1999).

As neither CBT, IPT, nor BWL is grounded in the affect regulation model, a new treatment based on remediating the hypothesized emotion regulation deficits in BN and BED was developed. DBT, originally developed by Linehan (1993a, 1993b), is the most comprehensive and empirically supported affect regulation treatment for borderline personality disorder to date (American Psychiatric Association, 2001). Among others, Telch (1997a, 1997b) recognized that DBT's conceptualization of self-injury as a functional (albeit maladaptive) affect regulation behavior in patients with borderline personality disorder might provide a helpful model for understanding the function (albeit maladaptive) of binge eating and/or purging as emotion regulation behaviors in patients with disordered eating. Given that DBT is specifically designed to teach adaptive affect regulation skills and to target behaviors resulting from affect dysregulation, a theoretical rationale exists for applying DBT to treat BED and BN (see also McCabe, La Via, & Marcus, 2004; Telch et al., 2000, 2001; Wisniewski & Kelly, 2003; Wiser & Telch, 1999).

RESEARCH EVIDENCE FOR DBT FOR BED AND BN

To date, preliminary studies investigating the adaptation of DBT to target disordered eating have been promising but limited to single case reports (Safer et al., 2001a; Telch, 1997b), uncontrolled case series (Palmer et al., 2003; Salbach-Andrae, Bohnekamp, Pfeiffer, Lehmkuhl, & Miller, 2008), uncontrolled trials (Salbach, Klinkowski, Pfeiffer, Lehmkuhl, & Korte, 2007; Telch et al., 2000), and three randomized controlled trials (Safer, Robinson, & Jo, in press; Safer et al., 2001b; Telch et al., 2001).

The treatment described in this book is currently the only adaptation of DBT for eating disorders that is supported through randomized trials in which clients were assigned, by chance, either to DBT as adapted for BED (Safer et al., in press; Telch et al., 2001) or BN (Safer et al., 2001b) or to a control condition (e.g., wait list or active nonspecific psychotherapy). Because factors that may influence outcome are distributed across groups randomly, the chance of a particular bias or factor confounding the results is minimized. Hence, randomized control trials are considered the most reliable form of scientific evidence for the efficacy of a clinical treatment (e.g., Chambless & Hollon, 1998).

This adapted DBT treatment was originally developed for adult women (ages 18–65) who met criteria for BED, BN, or partial BN (e.g., objective binge frequency = 1 episode/week for 3 months versus 2 episodes/week per DSM-IV-TR full criteria; American Psychiatric Association, 2000). Criteria by which individuals were excluded from entering the trials included (1) current use of psychotropic medications (Telch et al., 2001; Safer, Telch, & Agras, 2001b) or lack of a stable psychotropic dosage for the prior 3 months (Safer et al., in press); (2) psychotic or bipolar affective disorders diagnoses; (3) current involvement in psychotherapy or weight loss treatments; (4) current suicidality; (5) current substance abuse or dependence; or (6) pregnancy. Clients with borderline personality disorder were not specifically excluded, although only a few participants met full criteria for borderline personality disorder.

In the first randomized controlled trial of group DBT for BED, 89% (16 of 18) who completed DBT were abstinent from binge eating (e.g., had no objective binge episodes within the prior 4 weeks) by the end of the 20-week group treatment, compared with 12.5% (2 of 16) of individuals randomized to a wait list (Telch et al., 2001). The dropout rate was low. Of the original 22 assigned to DBT, only 9% (2 of 22) of those who attended at least the first session dropped out. At posttreatment, clients in DBT reported significantly improved weight and shape concerns, eating concerns, and, on the Emotional Eating Scale (Arnow et al., 1995), significantly reduced urges to eat when angry. At the 3-month and 6-month follow-up, 67% (12 of 18) and 56% (10 of 18), respectively, of the participants in DBT were abstinent from binge eating. DBT clients also reported practicing on average 3.6 different skills per week for an average of 4 days per week at the final assessment.

The high abstinence rates were consistent with those of a smaller uncontrolled trial of DBT for BED in which 82% of the participants were abstinent from binge eating after 20 group sessions, with none dropping out after commencing treatment (Telch et al., 2000). Similar findings were reported as part of a replication/ extension study of DBT for BED in which the client population was expanded to include both men and women and individuals on stable psychotropic medications (Safer et al., in press). Using a conservative statistical analysis that involved all participants, including those who dropped out from treatment (i.e., the intent-to-treat sample), the binge abstinence results for those receiving DBT for BED were 64% after 20 sessions, which was maintained at the 12-month follow-up (Safer et al., in press). These rates are similar to abstinence rates reported for CBT and IPT for BED by Wilfley et al. (1993, 2002). Long-term comparative studies are needed to clarify the relative response rates of particular participants to different treatment approaches.

In the randomized controlled trial of group DBT for BN, 20 weeks of individually delivered DBT for bulimic symptoms was compared with a wait-list control. Abstinence from binge-eating and purging behaviors at the end of 20 weeks of treatment was 28.6% (4 of 14) for DBT and 0% (0 of 15) for the wait-list control (Safer et al., 2001b). These findings were similar to posttreatment abstinence rates from the largest multisite CBT for BN trial (Agras, Walsh, Fairburn, Wilson, & Kraemer, 2000). Importantly, the effect sizes (which denote the magnitude of the effect of a treatment) showed that DBT resulted in moderate to large effect sizes for several of the emotion regulation measures, thus providing support for the role of decreasing affect dysregulation as a potential mechanism of DBT for BN. For example, on the Emotional Eating Scale (EES; Arnow et al., 1995), participants reported reduced urges to eat when angry, anxious, or depressed. In addition, the Positive and Negative Affect Schedule (Watson, Clark, & Tellegen, 1988) showed significant decreases in participants' experiences of negative affect. At posttreatment the dropout rate in DBT was 0%.

Such initial positive results provided the impetus, propelled by repeated requests from the clinical and research community, to provide a detailed description of how DBT was adapted to treat BED and the symptoms of BN. The result is this book, based on Telch's original manual (1997a). For those unfamiliar with standard DBT, the following chapter offers an orientation to standard DBT and to the adapted version for BED and BN.

CHAPTER 2

Orientation for Therapists

This chapter provides an orientation for therapists before they begin to implement treatment with clients. To provide context, we first describe the impetus behind this adapted DBT treatment's development. This is followed by a brief review of the empirical evidence for standard DBT. We then provide an introduction to this treatment model and assumptions and rationale that underlie this therapy, as well as its goals and targets. The final section of the chapter focuses on the delivery of this treatment, including basic therapist strategies and specifics regarding how sessions are structured.

IMPETUS FOR DEVELOPMENT OF THIS BOOK

The impetus for developing the treatment described in this book originated from years spent by one of us (C. F. T.) treating clients with eating disorders and conducting clinical research in this area. Part of this work included an ongoing search for more effective treatments for eating disorders. As discussed in Chapter 1, a sizable number of individuals with BED and BN do not receive maximum benefit from currently available psychotherapy treatments (e.g., CBT, IPT, BWL).

I reasoned that one potential explanation for this suboptimal treatment response may be a failure of such treatments to directly target the emotional aspects of binge eating. In other words, despite the considerable descriptive and experimental research supporting the relationship between emotional distress and disordered eating, neither CBT, IPT, nor BWL is based on an affect regulation model for binge eating.

In seeking more efficacious treatments for binge eating, I discovered a treatment developed by Marsha Linehan for individuals with borderline personality disorder: DBT. Standard DBT is based on the assumption that borderline personality disorder is best conceptualized as a dysfunction of the emotion regulation system such that many impulsive behaviors (e.g., suicidal behavior and nonsuicidal self-injury) are maladaptive attempts to regulate painful affects. As I investigated this treatment and received formal training in DBT, I became more convinced that the treatment model, principles, and strategies could be usefully adapted to treating individuals with eating disorders; thus the development and research that underlie this treatment manual.

In developing standard DBT, Linehan synthesized her clinical and research experience with BPD with principles and concepts from Western philosophy (dialectics), CBT, and both Eastern (Zen) and Western contemplative practices. DBT may be thought of as a synthesis of these divergent ideas and the application of this synthesis as a new means of treating emotional difficulties. DBT synthesizes a focus on both change and acceptance in the skills that are taught in the treatment.

Since originally developing standard DBT in the 1980s, Linehan (1993a, 1993b) standardized DBT into two manuals. These manuals, which describe the basics of dialectical philosophy, the therapeutic communication of both acceptance and change, and the core assumptions of DBT, should be read before applying the adapted treatment described in this book. As I worked to adapt DBT to eating disorders, I received extensive consultation from Linehan. With Linehan's permission, I "lifted" a great deal from Linehan's manuals and transplanted it into my original manual—*Emotion Regulation Skills Training Treatment for Binge Eating Disorder* (Telch, 1997a)—which serves as the basis for this book. Although each of the authors of this book has added her own thoughts and made modifications targeting the content of DBT to eating disorders, it is accepted that the adapted treatment presented is more or less an offspring of Linehan's manual. Therefore, Linehan's manuals are not cited each time material from them is used.

BRIEF REVIEW OF EMPIRICAL EVIDENCE FOR STANDARD DBT

Standard DBT is currently the most strongly empirically supported affect regulation treatment for borderline personality disorder (American Psychiatric Association, 2001) and is regarded as the treatment of choice for this disorder (Lieb, Zanarini, Schmahl, Linehan, & Bohus, 2004; Linehan, Comtois, et al., 2002). There are multiple randomized controlled trials of standard DBT to date (Linehan, Armstrong, Suarez, Allmon, & Heard, 1991; Linehan et al., 1999; Turner, 2000; Koons et al., 2001; Linehan, Dimeff, et al., 2002; Verheul et al., 2003; Linehan et al., 2006) and a number of nonrandomized controlled trials (Barley et al., 1993; Bohus et al., 2000; Stanley, Ivanoff, Brodsky, Oppenheim, & Mann, 1998; McCann, Ball, & Ivanoff, 2000; Rathus & Miller, 2002; Bohus, Haaf, & Simms, 2004).

With standard DBT, compared with treatment as usual (Linehan et al., 1991) or the more rigorous comparison of treatment by expert nonbehavioral therapists (Linehan et al., 2006), suicidal clients with borderline personality disorder (1) were significantly less likely to engage in suicidal behavior or nonsuicidal self-injury; (2) reported fewer episodes of suicidal behavior or nonsuicidal self-injury; (3) had less medically severe suicidal behavior or nonsuicidal self-injury; (4) were more likely to remain in treatment; (5) had fewer inpatient psychiatric days; (6) reported less anger; and (7) reported improved global and social adjustment at the end of treatment. All clients improved over time, with reduced symptoms of depression, hopelessness, and suicide ideation (Linehan et al., 1991; Linehan, Heard, & Armstrong, 1993; Linehan, Tutek, Heard, & Armstrong, 1994; Linehan et al., 2006). These findings were maintained at 1-year follow-up (Linehan et al., 2006).

Randomized controlled trials utilizing DBT for the treatment of borderline personality disorder and illicit substance use have also been efficacious (Linehan et al., 1999; Linehan, Dimeff, et al., 2002). Both of these studies demonstrated that participants assigned to DBT had significantly greater reductions in illicit substance use compared with a control treatment (Linehan et al., 1999; Linehan, Dimeff, et al., 2002).

INTRODUCTION TO TREATMENT MODEL, ASSUMPTIONS, AND RATIONALE

Before starting to work with clients using this treatment, therapists need to familiarize themselves with the basic definitions of emotion and emotion regulation as understood in DBT. Briefly, emotions are powerful biologically based reactions that organize our responses to internal and external stimuli. Emotions can be thought of as complex phenomena that affect the total response of an individual. Emotions have many "parts," including, but not limited to, the emotional experience (e.g., fear), the emotional expression (e.g., running), and the physiological activity (e.g., sweating). Although these basic components are shared, individuals will, of course, differ in (1) the intensity or strength of emotions; (2) the experience of positive and negative emotions; (3) emotional lability (i.e., how emotions fluctuate); and (4) the experience of particular emotions (e.g., shame, guilt). According to the DBT model, emotion regulation involves attempts by the individual to influence, change, or control emotions either by preventing an emotion from getting started (e.g., avoiding a feared situation) or by attempting to change the emotion once it has gotten under way (e.g., escaping a feared situation). Adaptive emotion regulation requires the ability to label, to monitor, and to modify emotional reactions, including the ability to accept and tolerate emotional experiences when emotions cannot, in the short run, be changed.

The theoretical model on which this treatment is based proposes that the core problem for individuals with BED and BN is emotion regulation dysfunction. This dysfunction is a result of both emotion vulnerability and inadequate skills for adaptive emotion regulation. That is, this model posits that a central and primary problem for these individuals involves deficits in labeling, monitoring, modifying, and accepting emotions.

Because individuals with BED and BN have underdeveloped emotion regulation skills, they frequently rely on maladaptive means, such as binge eating and/or purging, to control emotions. These behaviors may alter or influence emotions by distracting or suppressing emotional experience and expression, as well as by calming physiological arousal. The temporary relief provided strengthens the binge eating and/or purging as an emotion regulation strategy, and these behaviors become automatic, overlearned responses to emotion dysregulation, crowding out more adaptive strategies. Binge eating and/or purging behaviors are maladaptive because they are harmful to the individual in the long run, exacerbating maladaptive emotion regulation and profoundly interfering with physical, personal, and interpersonal health.

This treatment is also based on the assumption that the emotion regulation dysfunction evident in individuals with BED and BN is in part the result of emotional vulnerability. Emotional vulnerability is conceptualized as high sensitivity to emotional stimuli, intense emotional responding, and a slow return to emotional baseline. Individuals with BN report greater overall negative mood (Bulik et al., 1996; Waller et al., 2003), and individuals with BED (Greeno et al., 2000) report significantly more daily negative mood, as assessed on handheld computers, than those without BED. There is supporting research evidence (Masheb & Grilo, 2006) that individuals with BED and BN have emotion dysregulation across all emotions, including positive emotions such as joy and excitement. That is, binge eating and/or purging may be used to regulate strong feelings of excitement because, without adequate emotion regulation skills, the excitement is experienced as overwhelming and threatening. Finally, it is assumed that strong urges or impulses accompany emotions for individuals with BED and BN, as well as strong bodily reactions (e.g., increased heart rate). Therefore, without the requisite emotion regulation skills, individuals with BED and BN find it nearly impossible to refrain from acting on strong impulses to binge eat and/or purge in the face of emotional distress.

Role of Invalidating Environments

This treatment model assumes that the transaction over time between emotional vulnerability in individuals and the experience of a particular type of environment produces the emotion regulation deficits seen BED and BN. This particular environment is described as invalidating and is characterized by a tendency to respond negatively, inconsistently, and/or inappropriately to the individual's private experiences (e.g., beliefs, thoughts, feelings, and/or sensations). For example, to control the individual's behavior, crying may be met with nonresponsiveness, punishment, and/or criticism. Consequently, any expression of positive affect is not affirmed, validated, or attended to. In such environments, children learn that certain emotions and private experiences are unacceptable and dangerous because they lead to rejection, punishment, and disapproval.

The consequences of an invalidating environment during childhood development can include (1) the inability to label feelings, (2) an inability to trust one's own emotions as valid interpretations of events, (3) an inability to tolerate distress or adaptively regulate emotional arousal or emotional reactions, and (4) invalidation of one's own experience. Self-invalidation teaches one to mistrust one's internal states and to rely on the environment for clues on how to respond. This tendency to look for external validation leads to a failure to develop a sense of self. A core part of eating disorders is a preoccupation with external sources to dictate one's ideal weight and shape.

The rationale for teaching adaptive regulation skills to individuals with BED and BN should now be apparent. In order to stop using binge eating and/or purging to regulate emotions, these individuals need to learn adaptive emotion regulation skills that will replace the maladaptive binge eating. Otherwise, if such individuals stop binge eating and/or purging, another dysfunctional behavior may be substituted. This treatment also assumes that both acceptance and change skills are essential for adaptive emotion regulation.

Treatment Goals and Targets

The goals of treatment, the goals of skills training, and the targets of treatment are stated by the therapist in the pretreatment and first sessions and are outlined in a handout distributed during the first session (Chapter 3, Appendix 3.2). Refer to this material for further detail. Briefly, the primary goal of treatment is for clients to stop binge eating (and purging) and to stop all other problem eating behaviors listed in the target hierarchy (e.g., mindless eating, urges, cravings, capitulating to binge eating). The goals of treatment are accomplished by teaching the adaptive emotion regulation skills—Mindfulness skills, Emotion Regulation skills, and Distress Tolerance skills. Clients are taught to practice and use these adaptive Emotion Regulation skills to replace their maladaptive eating behaviors.

To accomplish these goals when we train our therapists, we teach them to focus on several key points. For example, we advise them to always "keep your eye on the prize"—that is, to remember that this treatment is aimed at stopping binge eating (and purging).[1] Therapists must be firm in their belief that binge eating is a serious maladaptive and destructive behavior that must stop altogether. Therapists are constantly on the lookout for any behaviors that even slightly resemble binge eating and work to help clients substitute the adaptive behaviors taught in the treatment for the problem eating behaviors.

Keeping your eye on the prize requires therapists constantly to link the client's goals of gaining control over eating behavior, specifically binge eating, with learning the skills. It is the therapists' job to convince clients that learning and practicing the Emotion Regulation skills taught in the treatment is critical to achieving their goals of stopping binge eating and gaining control over other problem behaviors. Additionally, it is imperative that therapists link the learning and practicing of the adaptive skills with an enhanced quality of life. That is, binge eating and problem eating behaviors produce guilt and shame and rob clients of their self-esteem and sense of mastery and competence.

Keeping your eye on the prize also requires therapists to adopt the notion of dialectical abstinence. This is described in the second session (Chapter 3, pp. 65–67). Briefly, the essence of dialectical abstinence is that therapists must, simultaneously, outwardly convey a firm conviction that each client in the program can and will stop binge eating while inwardly being poised and ready to "catch" clients when they fail and binge eat. Therapists must be absolutely certain that binge abstinence can be achieved and that clients can immediately stop binge eating at the start of the program. Therapists convey the attitude that this is essential and that there can be absolutely no middle ground. Clients must stop binge eating *now* in order to gain control over their lives. Of course, it is the therapists' job to help

---

[1]Although only binge eating is usually referred to throughout the remainder of the text, purging and any other compensatory behaviors (e.g., laxative abuse, fasting, overexercise)—when present—are always assumed to be an additional target.

clients figure out what to do in order to stop binge eating and to replace this behavior with adaptive behaviors, and, in this, therapists are very active in prescribing specific skills for clients to engage in to replace binge eating. Therapists provide the momentum, the conviction, the "jump start" until clients can continue this movement on their own. On the other hand, therapists are simultaneously ready to "pick clients up" when they fail. Therapists help clients learn how to fail well. That is, although therapists convey the conviction that clients can and must stop binge eating, therapists nonjudgmentally accept clients who fall short of this and engage in binge eating. Therapists respond to binge eating by acknowledging that binge abstinence is hard while maintaining the conviction that the client can achieve it. After a client breaks binge abstinence, therapists explain that the task now is to accept the disappointment, learn from the failure, and commit from this moment on to repair the self-harm done by never again binge eating.

Keeping your eye on the prize requires attention to the number-one treatment target listed on the target hierarchy—to stop any behavior that interferes with treatment. Therapists are clear with clients that they believe that binge eating and problem eating behaviors will not stop without treatment. Therefore, because the clients' goals are to stop binge eating and to gain control over their eating and their lives, clients must receive treatment to achieve these goals. If clients are not in treatment, they are less likely to get better. Any behavior that interferes with receiving treatment (e.g., absences, late arrivals) are top priority, and therapists, at the onset of treatment, elicit a commitment from clients to address any treatment-interfering behaviors. Once this is made clear, therapists do not need to refer to this again unless treatment-interfering behavior arises.

Within our research trials, a final requirement of keeping your eye on the prize has been that therapists adhere to the treatment protocol described in this book. For example, at the trials run at Stanford, we emphasized to therapists that teaching the skills prescribed is absolutely nonnegotiable. What is negotiable is how they are taught. That is, the strategies used to present them must be employed flexibly. Therapists must decide, when delivering the treatment, whether or not a particular strategy is appropriate to use given the context of what is taking place in the session. For example, the book may suggest using the devil's advocate strategy to enhance client commitment, but given the context of that particular group, Extending may be more appropriate. The strategies or tools used to teach the skills are negotiable and therefore may be used flexibly.

It is important to point out that clients, particularly those with BED, will likely express concern about whether or not treatment is aimed at losing weight. Therapists must validate that this is an understandable concern, one that is shared by the therapists, who are also concerned about the client's weight to the extent that excess weight reflects maladaptive eating behaviors. However, therapists must make clear that this is not specifically a weight loss program in that diet, nutrition, and meal prescriptions are not a treatment focus. It is assumed that clients who learn and use the adaptive skills for regulating emotions taught in treatment will stop binge eating and gain increased control over their eating in general, and as a result their weight may decrease (also see Chapter 3). Clients are asked to monitor their weight weekly to allow evaluation of any changes in weight that coincide with treatment.

DELIVERING THE TREATMENT: BASIC THERAPIST STRATEGIES

DBT for BED/BN utilizes the same treatment strategies as standard DBT (Linehan, 1993a, 1993b). These include its use of dialectical strategies (e.g., balancing validation and change, modeling dialectical thinking), problem-solving and solution-analysis strategies (e.g., chain analysis), stylistic strategies (e.g., irreverence), commitment strategies (e.g., Evaluating Pros and Cons, Playing Devil's Advocate, Foot in the Door, Door in the Face, Connecting Present Commitments to Prior Commitments, Highlighting Freedom to Choose in the Absence of Alternatives, and Cheerleading), structural strategies, and treatment team consultation strategies (e.g., weekly meetings of therapists).

These treatment strategies are described briefly here and given greater detail at relevant points in subsequent chapters.

Dialectical Strategies

DBT is based on a dialectical worldview that stresses the fundamental interrelatedness or wholeness of reality and connects the immediate to the larger contexts of behavior. From a dialectical worldview, reality is not seen as static but as comprising opposing forces (thesis and antithesis) out of which synthesis can evolve, generating a new set of opposing forces. The individual is stuck in polarities, unable to move beyond the conflict, and the therapist assists the client to resolve the dialectical dilemma or conflict and move to a synthesis. The synthesis is a different way of being, a different perspective that moves beyond the conflict. From this viewpoint, the fundamental dialectical strategy used by therapists is to stay aware of the polarities the client is stuck in and suggest ways out (e.g., use of skills).

The primary dialectical strategy for therapists to focus on when delivering this treatment is the balance between acceptance and change. The essential "attitude" of therapists that pervades this treatment is one of sensitivity to the balance between the need for clients to accept themselves just as they are and the need for them to change. This dialectic is clearly represented by the concept of dialectical abstinence. The guiding principle of dialectics is also reflected in the skills taught, including both Radical Acceptance and Loving You Emotion—in addition to skills for changing emotions. The therapist must both accept and validate the current circumstances of the individual while simultaneously teaching behavioral skills that deliver the message that things must change.

The therapist balances pushing the client toward change in order to have a better life and holding the client with an acceptance of how the client is in the moment. In this context, the therapist must be acutely aware of the client's tendency toward imbalance in either leaning too far toward pushing for change or not changing despite change being needed. It is the job of the therapist to provide the balance. The aim is to help clients become comfortable with change and to accept change as part of reality.

The dialectical attitude toward acceptance and change is conveyed in part by the therapist's balanced application of both validation and problem-solving strategies. The essence of validation is the communication that a response is understandable in the current context. Given the current set of circumstances and the client's learning history and belief structure, the therapist recognizes and communicates that the client's response makes sense and is valid. Validation is not sugarcoating, whitewashing, or reassuring. For example, if the client claims: "I'm so stupid to have let my boss get to me so that I ended up going home and binge eating after work," validating this client would not mean saying, "You're not stupid." Validating would involve acknowledging the client's experience of feeling stupid, commenting that it is both understandable that the client responded as she or he did and that she or he feels stupid in hindsight. Validating does not include validating the invalid. So in this case the therapist would not want to validate binge eating as an effective response to emotional distress.

In a nutshell, a dialectical treatment approach (1) searches for synthesis and balance to replace the rigid and dichotomous responses characteristic of dysfunctional individuals and (2) enhances clients' comfort with ambiguity and change, which are viewed as inevitable aspects of life.

Of the many dialectical strategies (see also Linehan, 1993a, Ch. 7, pp. 199–220), two others noted here are Extending and Making Lemonade Out of Lemons. In Extending, which is based on aikido, the therapist stays with a client rather than opposing him or her and then takes the client one step further so that the client is thrown off balance and is more open to new direction. The essence of Making Lemonade Out of Lemons is making opportunities out of difficult situations. As Winston Churchill reportedly said, "The pessimist sees the difficulty in every opportunity. The optimist sees the opportunity in every difficulty." It is important to convey that one can learn from mistakes. For example, individuals with BED and BN often feel demoralized and filled with shame after a binge, with a tendency to avoid thinking about the episode. In such an instance, the therapist acknowledges the "lemons" while also utilizing the experience as an opportunity to understand the antecedents to the problem behavior and to identify effective skills to be employed next time. Therapists should look for multiple opportunities to employ this strategy and help clients learn to pick themselves up from "failures" by turning the failures into learning experiences.

Problem-Solving and Solution-Analysis Strategies

Problem-solving strategies involve a two-stage process of, first, accepting that there is a problem and, second, generating alternative adaptive responses. This means that the therapist first helps the client to observe and describe in a nonjudgmental manner the problematic binge-eating and impulsive-behavior patterns. Second, following the nonjudgmental analysis of the problem eating behavior, the therapist helps the client to generate alternative effective and adaptive solutions. This involves identifying skills that have been taught and working on client motivation to use the skills.

Problem-solving and solution-analysis strategies are woven throughout this treatment and involve a detailed examination of the problem behavior accompanied by the generation of alternative adaptive responses. The use of a detailed chain-analysis monitoring form in this treatment (see Chapter 3, Appendix 3.6) helps clients to identify the events and factors leading up to and following the targeted problem behavior. The solution analysis involves the identification of alternative adaptive responses (i.e., identifying skills to use). The chain-analysis monitoring form is completed by the client for each instance of targeted problem behaviors and reported on during the homework review section of the session.

Stylistic Strategies

Therapists conducting this treatment balance a responsive and empathic communication style conveying warmth and understanding with an irreverent style delivered in a matter-of-fact manner. One or the other is used moment to moment in sessions, depending on what the situation calls for. Responsive, empathic communication is usually most appropriate when assisting the client to accept him- or herself and to help him or her to move out of negative self-judging. The matter-of-fact communication is a strategy to help get a client who seems unable to see things from a different perspective to become "unstuck." The irreverent communication strategy is designed to gently shock or wake the client up by being quite frank and honest with her or him, thus helping the client to get moving. For example, if a client says "I couldn't keep practicing the skills because they were taking too much time," the therapist, with a humorous tone, may say, "Ah—I get it. Practicing the skills took up too much time ... but you *were* able to fit in time for a binge," or "If you had time to binge, you had time to practice the skills."

Motivation and Commitment Strategies

Eliciting commitment and agreements from clients is an ongoing task for therapists throughout treatment. The first agreement clients make is to come to treatment. The next is to agree that the goal of treatment is to stop binge eating, and the next is to learn and practice the skills. Therapists constantly gauge a client's level of commitment, using motivation and commitment strategies as commitment waxes and wanes.

In DBT, motivation is not viewed as an internal state or an intrinsic quality of the client. Instead, therapists understand the necessary role of situational variables that, when present, increase the likelihood that clients will exhibit a desired behavior (i.e., be "motivated"). Therapists also keep in mind that eliciting commitment and agreement from a client is an ongoing job that requires therapists to constantly gauge the client's current level of commitment, returning to the motivation and commitment strategies as the client's commitment waxes and wanes.

In standard DBT, group skills training focuses on remediating clients' deficits in capability, whereas individual treatment helps clients identify applications of the newly taught skills to everyday situations and also involves analyzing motivational issues that may interfere. This analyzing may take the form of a behavioral chain analysis or a solution analysis, or it may involve using commitment strategies.

The challenge for therapists conducting this adapted DBT treatment is to provide in one session both the motivational component usually focused on during individual treatment in standard DBT and the skills training usually taught in group skills training (see also Chapter 3). It is the job of therapists to cheerlead clients in using skills in difficult situations. When clients give up, the therapist should not assume that clients either can or cannot solve problems for themselves.

Wherever possible, the therapist needs to work on "dragging out" new behaviors in clients in these situations.

Commitment strategies are discussed briefly here and throughout the relevant sections of this book. Again, readers are also referred to Linehan's text (1993a, particularly pp. 284–291) as essential reading. Evaluating Pros and Cons involves helping the client review the advantages of whatever behavior is being evaluated, as well as counterarguments to those advantages. The therapist should highlight the short- and long-term consequences of the pros and cons. For example, behaviors that look attractive in the short run may have very negative sequelae. In Playing the Devil's Advocate, the therapist counters or challenges the client in a way that results in the client's providing his or her own reasons that he or she *must* change. In the Foot-in-the-Door technique (Freedman & Fraser, 1966), the therapist enhances compliance by first asking for something easy, followed by something more difficult. In the Door-in-the-Face techniques (Cialdini et al., 1975), the therapist first makes a challenging request followed by an easier one. In Connecting Present Commitments to Prior Commitments, the therapist reminds the client of previously made commitments to bolster a commitment that may be waning or when the client is behaving in ways that are inconsistent with previous commitments. The strategy of Highlighting Freedom to Choose in the Absence of Alternatives enhances commitment by emphasizing the client's choice to do whatever he or she wishes while highlighting the lack of effective alternatives.

Treatment Team Consultation Strategies

The primary strategy here is a weekly meeting of therapists. The purposes of these team consultation meetings are (1) to review and evaluate adherence to the protocol; (2) to "treat the therapist" by providing a nonjudgmental environment for each therapist to observe and describe his or her own behavior, thoughts, and feelings regarding the week's sessions and for other team members to provide nonjudgmental feedback, validation, and suggestions for change; and (3) to discuss how best to handle any therapy-interfering behaviors on the part of any group members or clients receiving individual therapy.

Structural Strategies

Treatment is structured or organized around the specific targets outlined in the treatment target hierarchy (Chapter 3, Appendix 3.2). The targets include both problem eating behaviors that must stop and the skills that must be learned in order to accomplish this. By orienting clients to the skills being taught and how to use them, the therapist bridges the gap between the client's goal of stopping binge eating and the client's learning of the new skills. For example, the therapist might say: "OK—so this is what you can do when you're feeling depressed if you don't want to feel that way. Opposite action means doing the opposite of what your mood is telling you to do. So the opposite of depression—which tells you to withdraw and to stay inactive—is getting active." Therapists give clear instructions as to how clients can apply the skills being taught rather than assuming that clients possess this ability.

STRUCTURE OF GROUP SESSIONS

As described briefly, this adapted treatment combines elements of the functions of two distinct modalities in standard DBT: individual psychotherapy (enhancement of motivation) and group skills training (acquisition/strengthening of new skills).[2] With much to accomplish, each 2-hour weekly group session should start on time, whether or not all group members are present. Therapists begin by greeting the group. If a group member arrives late or has missed a previous session, she or he is asked to briefly state what occurred as part of her or his turn during the homework review. This attention to behavior that interferes with receiving treatment is very important, and absences or late arrivals should not be ignored. But after this brief attention, therapists should move on. If a group member is not present and is expected, one of the cotherapists may call to check in and encourage the client to attend the group. With clients who are repeatedly absent or late, group leaders should use their judgment and may wish to address this privately with the group member in a brief phone call or an in-person meeting. If necessary, a chain analysis will be performed targeting this therapy-interfering behavior.

Homework Review: Diary Cards and Chain Analyses

Chapter 3 discusses the structure of the homework review in greater detail. Briefly, the first half of each session (50 minutes for group sessions, 25 minutes for individual sessions) is devoted to a review of the past week's skills practice and chain analyses conducted on targeted behaviors. In the group format, each group member should have about 5 minutes to report on her or his use of the new skills and to describe specific successes or difficulties in applying the skills to replace problem eating behaviors. The therapists check with each group member to make sure she or he can explain what skills were used, how she or he used them, and whether they were effective. Group members should be encouraged to help one another identify solutions to problems encountered in applying the skills and to "cheerlead" the efforts each fellow group member makes.

Therapists clearly convey that each group member will be asked about her or his skills practice and that the member will be questioned about skills not practiced. This serves to motivate clients to use the skills at some point during the week so as to have something to share. Clearly stating that each member will be asked to share each week sets the norm for practice and can be a source of motivation. Therapists should be alert to the possibility of a group member feeling "stu-

---

[2]Although our data are based on the structure used in our research trials, wherein BED treatment was delivered over 20 weekly 2-hour group sessions and BN treatment over 20 weekly 50-minute individual format sessions, there are no data to suggest that changing the delivery method would adversely affect clinical outcomes. Indeed, Telch's case report (1997b) demonstrated good response in a client with BED receiving treatment via individual sessions. Therefore, therapists treating individuals with BED or BN may administer the treatment in either a group or individual format. Similarly, although our research studies tested 20 treatment sessions, differences between research and clinic settings may require therapists to cover the material at a different rate. Chapters 3–7 focus on the skills to be taught, not on the time allotted for the therapist to teach them. For therapists wishing to replicate our studies, the appendix to this book outlines the specific content covered in each session.

pid," ashamed, or embarrassed about sharing and can discuss which of the skills would be useful to practice in this circumstance.

Because a very limited amount of time is available, therapists should help clients to be very focused. Chapter 3 offers more guidance. Briefly, clients are asked to report on two items. The first is a report of their practice of the skills during the prior week and their use of skills to replace maladaptive binge eating and other problem eating behaviors. The basis for this sharing about skills practice is the diary card, which each client is expected to have completed. The second item is the client's report on the chain analysis conducted on the targeted eating behaviors. Each client reports on the target behavior highest in the hierarchy (Chapter 3, Appendix 3.2). For example, if binge eating and/or purging—the highest targets— occurred, the client must report on the chain analysis of that behavior. If binge eating and/or purging occurs, it is important for therapists to keep in mind the concept of dialectical abstinence (Chapter 3) to help clients fail effectively so that they can get back up and make a commitment to never binge again from this moment on. If binge eating and/or purging did not occur, the next target on the hierarchy would be discussed.

In the homework review, the client is asked to report on (1) a key dysfunctional link identified on the path to the problematic behavior (see Chapter 3 for details) and (2) what skill or skills they could have used and will try to use next time to replace that dysfunctional link.

For clients having difficulty with skills practice and application, therapists need to assess the nature of that difficulty. For example, first determine whether the problem is due to a lack of understanding of the skill, to a lack of skill practice, or to motivational factors. If the problem is due to a lack of understanding, a brief review—ideally offered by another group member—may be indicated. If the client understands the skill, determine whether greater strengthening is needed through additional practice. If so, help the client to set realistic practice goals. If the problem is due to a lack of motivation, the commitment strategies described earlier and given in greater detail in Chapter 3 (and see also Linehan, 1993a) are utilized. For instance, the therapist may have the client review pros and cons of practicing skills, form a plan of action to practice skills, and commit to the plan to overcome obstacles to skills practice (including self-criticism for lack of practice) for the upcoming week. Therapists must be careful not to join in punishing or criticizing the client but help her or him to recommit to practice. Therapists should describe and validate any successes described, as well as failures. This may mean validating how difficult it can be to use the skills under extremely stressful conditions. If therapists are judgmental about group members' difficulties, clients may feel free to share only successes.

Therapists may suggest to clients who repeatedly fail to practice the skills that they use the chain analysis form to analyze this problem. In other words, lack of skills practice is the targeted problem (treatment-interfering behavior) analyzed in detail via a chain analysis. Conducting a chain analysis is a skilled behavior in and of itself, and helping clients to develop this skill is key to adaptive behavior.

Therapists must search for and praise every small approximation of using the skills. For example, therapists can distinguish between the client's attempts to use the skills and the outcome. Praise should be offered for effort, followed by helping the client analyze what happened, what interfered, and how the client can be more effective with the use of skills the next time.

Therapists should watch for any clients who always use the same skill. In such cases, remind clients that the objective is to develop the ability to use each skill. Once a skill is learned, clients can choose not to use it. But experience with all the skills allows clients to make informed decisions about whether or not a particular skill is best for them given the circumstances.

In summary, problems that come up in the homework review can be addressed by briefly:

1. Formulating hypotheses about the possible factors involved in producing the problem behavior.
2. Generating skills solutions by asking, "What skills could you have used here?"
3. Encouraging group members to commit to trying out the skills solutions suggested.

In our research setting, at the end of the review of skills practice, therapists collect any diary cards, homework sheets, chain analyses, and so forth.

Break

During 2-hour group sessions, a 5- to 8-minute break should take place after the homework review to allow group members to use the restroom, get a drink of water, stretch, and so forth. Inform the group members that the second half of the session will begin promptly to allow a full hour during which instruction and practice of the new skills can take place.

Skills Instruction

In general, teaching each skill involves:

1. Providing an explanation or rationale for including the skill in this treatment program—that is, explaining to clients why this skill is being taught, why it is important, and how it is relevant to clients' goals of stopping binge eating and gaining control over problem eating behaviors.
2. Skill acquisition—describing the skill and specific steps for learning the skill.
3. Skill strengthening—demonstrating how to practice the skill and providing opportunities to practice that skill during the group sessions.
4. Skill generalization—providing suggestions for using skills during daily life. Therapists should enlist clients in generating ideas about how skills can be used to replace binge eating and other problem behaviors when emotions are dysregulated.

The teaching of skills is facilitated by the use of handouts and homework materials. The idea is to make learning the skills relevant to clients' lives. To make sure group members are active and involved in the discussion, therapists should ask questions that check for skill comprehension and to enlist ideas for skill utilization. To facilitate comprehension, therapists should focus on making a few key points, using the remainder of the time to illustrate with metaphors and stories, to reinforce, or simply to rephrase those key points.

At the end of the session, therapists should clarify and review the homework for the upcoming week. This involves describing homework sheets and making sure clients understand how to practice and record the skills. Then, during the session's final minutes, a wind-down is offered. This involves a few minutes of practicing a specific skill (e.g., diaphragmatic breathing).

In conclusion, there is a great deal to cover in each session, with very little time to do so. Therapists must therefore be flexible, using skillful means to be effective rather than trying to be perfect. When necessary, therapists must be willing to give up making each and every point during instruction of a skill if the situation calls for spending more time on a client's question. Alternatively, if the therapist feels the skills training will suffer as a result of omitting a point, the therapist might offer to discuss the question over the break. The idea is to always keep one's eye on the prize—helping clients stop binge eating by teaching adaptive skills when emotions are dysregulated.

CHAPTER 3

The Pretreatment Stage

The Pretreatment Interview and Introductory Sessions

This chapter describes how the pretreatment stage is conceptualized and structured in DBT for BED or BN. The overall goals of this stage are to (1) orient the client to treatment, (2) obtain the client's agreement to treatment, and (3) obtain the client's commitment to abstinence from binge eating (and purging). In our research, this stage begins after we complete the diagnostic assessments and determine the client to be eligible for entry into the study.

When treatment is conducted in a group format, the orientation stage includes (1) a pregroup pretreatment interview (conducted individually with each group member in the 1–2 weeks prior to the start of the group) and (2) introductory sessions conducted in the group format. In our research studies of 20 sessions, these introductory sessions usually are covered during the first 2 weeks of treatment. When therapy takes place in an individual-session format, a pretreatment interview is also necessary. One of the goals of the pretreatment interview—obtaining a commitment to coming to treatment—is essential to establish before obtaining a commitment to stop binge eating and/or purging. The purpose of the next session, what we term the introductory session, is a more involved elicitation of a verbal commitment to stop binge eating (and purging). However, if constraints of a particular clinic setting are such that a separate pretreatment session is not feasible, the pretreatment interview goals and materials may be combined in an initial session, with the commitment to treatment attendance a prerequisite to addressing the commitment to abstinence from binge eating (and purging). Nonetheless, it is our experience that separating the functions of the pretreatment and introductory material into distinct sessions is desirable when conducting treatment in an individual-session format, as this gives the therapist adequate time to underscore the importance of the commitments and the treatment without feeling rushed and potentially covering the material in a cursory fashion.

THE PRETREATMENT INTERVIEW

The pretreatment interview has a number of important and specific goals. Usually requiring 30–45 minutes, it is not intended to replace a standard clinical intake (e.g., history of present illness, past psychiatric and medical history, social history) but is scheduled after such diagnostic assessment has been completed. The goals of the pretreatment interview are presented here and discussed in greater detail in the relevant subsections in this chapter, as well as in the case examples in Chapter 8.

Goals of the Pretreatment Interview

The seven goals of the pretreatment interview follow.

1. Develop a therapeutic alliance.
2. Gain an understanding of the client's overall eating difficulties.
3. Provide clients with a rationale for DBT treatment.
4. Orient clients to treatment and obtain commitment.
5. Review treatment expectations for the client and the therapist.
6. Provide logistical information and opportunity for questions.
7. Convey enthusiasm.

Especially in settings in which the diagnostic assessment has been conducted by a member of the team other than the therapist (e.g., research assistant, study physician), the pretreatment interview may be the first opportunity for the therapist to actually meet the client. The most important goal of this meeting is for the therapist (or cotherapist when treatment is in a group format) to begin to develop a therapeutic alliance. The second goal of the pretreatment interview is to provide the therapist with an opportunity to gain a general picture of the client's difficulties with eating. In the case of Sarah, age 36, in Chapter 8, her binge eating and purging tended to occur during evenings when her husband traveled and she had been particularly stressed supervising her two children's homework and getting them ready for bed.

The third goal is to provide a rationale for the treatment the client is about to commence. This involves introducing the client to the Emotion Dysregulation Model of Problem Eating (Appendix 3.1), with the therapist assessing the model's personal relevance and fit for the client.

The fourth goal involves orienting the client to the treatment's goals and targets and obtaining the client's commitment to these. This includes a discussion of the concept of treatment-interfering behavior (e.g., not coming to therapy). Obtaining a commitment to treatment attendance sets the stage for addressing treatment-interfering behaviors should they emerge. The fifth goal is to review treatment expectations for both the client and the therapist. These are listed in Appendices 3.3–3.5. The sixth goal is to provide practical information, such as the dates and times of treatment, and to give the client an opportunity to ask questions. Typical questions posed by clients are described later. The seventh and a final goal of the pretreatment interview is to provide the therapist with the opportunity to convey enthusiasm about the start of treatment and the client's participation. The therapist's conviction about the value of the treatment and confidence in the client's ability to succeed increase the chance of a constructive start to treatment—filled with positive expectations and hopefulness.

Orienting the Client to the Pretreatment Interview and Dates of Treatment

Therapists begin the pretreatment interview by introducing themselves. Make sure to express enthusiasm even during this first meeting, perhaps saying something such as: "I'm very happy you'll be joining us. We're all so excited about this treatment approach." Explain that the purpose of the pretreatment interview is to get to know the client and to provide an overview of the treatment program, as discussed later.

From the outset, it is important to underscore the link between commitment to the course of treatment and the client's ability to overcome her or his binge eating (and purging) behaviors. For example, the therapist might say:

> "We know that it is very important to you to stop binge eating [and purging] and to gain control over your eating behaviors. Your accomplishing these goals is very important to us, too. One thing we assume is that if you could change these behaviors on your own, you would have done so by now. To give this treatment a chance to work, you'll need the full course. It is crucial to commit to coming to each session even when you don't feel like it—especially then!—or it is particularly inconvenient. You might think about it as being prescribed a certain amount of antibiotics to take if you're ill. It is important to take the whole dose, even if some days you don't feel like it or are feeling as if you don't need it. It takes a lot of effort to stop binge eating [and purging], and we want you to succeed, so receiving a full dose of the treatment is important."

Discussing Dates of Treatment and Making Up Missed Sessions

During the pretreatment interview, the therapist should review the client's availability for the scheduled period of treatment. In our research studies, clients, during the assessment period, compared their schedules with the dates of scheduled sessions. Clients who, at the outset of treatment, determined that they would have to miss more than three group sessions were unfortunately not able to join the group.[1] Of course, in individual treatment, scheduling can be more flexible, but every attempt should still be made to keep treatment as continuous as possible, with missed sessions rescheduled quickly. If sessions are carried out in a group format and are recorded on audio or video, the therapist explains at this juncture (to be revisited as needed subsequently) that clients who cannot avoid missing sessions (e.g., due to illness) are required to set up a time to make up the missed material by coming to listen to the recordings.

---

[1]This differs from standard DBT (Linehan, 1993b, p. 23), in which clients who miss 4 weeks of scheduled skills training sessions in a row are dropped from treatment.

Asking about the Client's Prior Treatment Experience

We recommend inquiring about the client's prior therapy experiences. The therapist might say, "I am going to give you a general idea of the treatment, but first I'd like to learn more about you. Have you been in a group before? Have you been in one like this? If yes, what did you like or did not like? Are there any issues you foresee?" In our experience, it was not unusual for clients to have obtained support for their eating concerns through such groups as Overeaters Anonymous, Weight Watchers support groups, and/or therapist-led groups. Therapists may wish to emphasize, particularly if clients report a negative past experience with such groups, the differences between this current treatment approach (i.e., a structured, skills-based group with an eating-disorder focus) and what they have tried. We also try to help clients cope ahead of time with any reported difficulties they have experienced with past treatment attempts.

Introducing the Emotion Dysregulation Model

We have found it helpful to introduce the emotion dysregulation model of problem eating (i.e., binge eating and/or purging; Appendix 3.1) by having the client describe a typical problematic eating episode and using this as a basis for assessing the model's personal relevance and fit for the client. The therapist might commence as follows: "Now I would like to ask you about a recent or typical binge [and purge]. Can you describe in as much detail as possible what was going on for you at the time? What circumstances preceded the binge [and purge]? What feelings were you having?"

Following the client's description, the therapist presents the emotion dysregulation model of problem eating (see Appendix 3.1) and uses particulars from what the client has revealed to describe the flow of events.

During the discussion, the therapist looks for opportunities to make the following points:

• "This model assumes that emotions are reactions to internal or external events. In other words, something in your environment, such as an argument, and/or something in yourself, such as your thinking, triggers an emotion or set of emotions."

• "Emotions, whether they are negative emotions such as sadness or anger or positive emotions like happiness or joy, can be uncomfortable. Feeling any emotion too strongly or too intensely can be difficult and therefore requires skillful emotion regulation."

• "An assumption of this model [and one that seems to be accurate based on what I'm hearing from your description of the binge ...] is that you have not developed the means and are therefore frequently ill equipped to manage your emotional experience. At least at times, you just don't have the skills you need to tolerate how you feel."

• "Furthermore, because of all the times you've turned to food in the past, you have a *low expectancy* that you can handle your emotions any other way than through using food. So you have uncomfortable emotions, and you don't believe you can handle them or soothe yourself."

• "You've come to believe that the only option you have is binge eating [and purging] as a way of coping with your emotions. It becomes a sort of automatic, overlearned behavior."

• "Temporarily, binge eating [and purging] may lead to a decrease in the distress by giving you a way to avoid how you feel, a means of escaping for the moment. You don't have to face your emotions or put in an effort to cope with them because the food serves to distract you."

• "In the short term, binge eating [and purging] works to 'solve the problem' of managing uncomfortable emotions. But in the long run, which is why you've come for treatment, there is a high cost. For example, binge eating [and purging] often leads to feeling guilt and shame, which can lead to more binge eating [and purging] and feeling hopeless. Your self-confidence is diminished and your expectation that you can handle difficult feelings is further eroded."

• "Skillful emotion regulation behaviors include the ability to monitor, evaluate, and modify your emotional reactions. They also include the ability to accept and tolerate emotional experiencing when nothing can be changed immediately. These adaptive emotional coping skills may reduce the experience of an emotion before it starts in the first place and may modify the behavioral expression of an emotion that has been experienced. Overall, the goal is to manage your emotional experiences and behaviors in a way that leads to achieving your life goals."

• "This treatment will help you express emotions and enable you to live your life without using food as a solution to emotional distress. We also assume that some problems can't be solved, but that it's better to live with the problem than to turn to a destructive solution. In this treatment you will learn to replace your maladaptive responses with adaptive emotion regulation strategies."

After making the preceding points, the therapist asks questions to facilitate the client's beginning to incorporate the model and rationale into his or her thinking. For example: "What do you think of this model and the assumptions of this treatment? Does it seem to fit for you? Are there ways in which it does not make sense?"

Orienting the Client to the Goals of Treatment, Goals of Skills Training, and Treatment Targets Handout

Once the client understands the treatment model, the therapist can review the Goals of Treatment, Goals of Skills Training, and Treatment Targets handout (Appendix 3.2). It is essential for the therapist to link the client's goals and the treatment targets to the learning and practicing of the skills. For example, the therapist might point out:

> "What is really important to you and the reason you joined this program is that you want to stop binge eating [and purging]. If you just stopped binge eating [and purging] without developing skillful means to cope with your emotions,

another dysfunctional, maladaptive behavior could emerge in the place of binge eating [and purging]. The basic premise of this treatment program is that by learning and practicing adaptive and skillful ways to cope with your emotions, you can use the skills to replace your maladaptive binge eating [and purging], other problem eating behaviors, and other maladaptive means you currently use to cope with your emotions. This treatment focuses on helping you acquire, strengthen, and apply adaptive skills for gaining emotional control to eliminate the need to rely on strategies such as binge eating [and purging]."

Sarah, for example, the harried mother of two, would become more aware of her emotional state by observing muscle tension in her back and shoulders.

The therapist begins at the top of the handout, reading and discussing each point. The client's agreement and commitment to each major aspect of the treatment is elicited before moving on. In our experience, the client's commitment to the treatment goals and targets during the pretreatment interview is, for the most part, straightforwardly obtained. For example, after the therapist orients the client to the goals of treatment (e.g., saying, "In this treatment, the primary goal is to stop binge eating [and purging]. This is the top priority. The goal also includes control over other problem eating behaviors, as I'll describe," and asking, "But first, do you agree with this overall goal?"), we have found it very likely that clients in our treatment studies will readily agree. However, some clients may be hesitant. If it seems helpful, reassure them that although they need to be 100% certain of the goal to stop binge eating (and purging), they may simultaneously be uncertain about their ability to accomplish this goal. Here is where therapy and learning the skills will help the clients out. These are the means by which they will meet their goals.

In DBT for BED or BN (as in standard DBT), commitment is viewed as a process, a behavior to be elicited, learned, and reinforced. In the pretreatment interview, the therapist first and foremost is encouraging a commitment to treatment. The commitment to the treatment targets and goals is also encouraged and strengthened during the first introductory session.

When attempting to secure a commitment to the goals of skills training regarding learning and practicing the skills, the therapist might explain, "The goal of skills training is to learn and practice adaptive emotion regulation skills." The therapist will be satisfied and move on if the client agrees when asked: "Does this make sense to you? Do you agree to this goal?" For most clients, the orientation to the emotion dysregulation model of problem eating is sufficiently relevant to the client's understanding of his or her problematic eating that a goal of learning skillful emotion regulation behaviors is logical.

Orienting the Client to the Path to Mindful Eating

The therapist explains, "We call this the 'path to mindful eating.' By 'mindful eating,' we mean eating with awareness, in the present moment. Mindful eating is the opposite of binge eating—which is eating without awareness or a sense of control." In order to help clients effectively achieve the capacity to eat mindfully, the following treatment hierarchy has been established. At the top of that hierarchy is stopping any behavior that interferes with the client's ability to receive treatment.

Stopping Any Behavior That Interferes with Treatment

Highlight the idea that any behavior that interferes with participating effectively in treatment will be the top priority of treatment. The therapist might explain:

> "I know you've committed to stopping binge eating as your overall goal. At the same time, if you are not feeling like coming to sessions, if you are missing sessions, are not doing your homework or are not practicing the skills—these issues would need to addressed first. You are learning how to stop binge eating, and we both know that if you could have done this on your own, you would not be here. So, part of our job together is to identify anything that is getting in the way of treatment and to work on it. How can you learn the skills if you're not here, right? Can you agree to that, that this is the top target on your path to mindful eating?"

Stopping Binge Eating (and Purging)

The therapist explains, "When we talk about binge eating, we are referring to eating a large or small amount of food in which the predominant experience is being out of control." The therapist makes reference to the previously discussed "typical binge" used to illustrate the emotion dysregulation model of binge eating. The behaviors of purging and/or other compensatory behaviors (e.g., using laxatives or diuretics, fasting, overexercising) are targeted here, too. The therapist might say, "Stopping these behaviors is essential to gain an improved quality of life. Do you agree with that goal?" In our experience, most clients nod in agreement with this goal despite admitting some nervousness. After obtaining agreement, the therapist then explains that the remaining behaviors are targeted because they are believed to set clients up to binge eat (and purge).

Eliminating Mindless Eating

Define mindless eating as eating without the awareness that one is eating, or eating on "automatic pilot." This includes overeating or eating when one is not physically hungry and is not paying attention (such as when watching television). Mindless eating can also involve chaotic eating, such as snacking throughout the evening because one has not planned a meal. Mindless eating is not equivalent to binge eating, because it does not entail the experience of a loss of control. However, mindless eating frequently leads to binge eating (and purging). For example, mindless eating would involve a client noticing, after the fact, that a whole bowl of chips has been emptied without recalling having eaten them—prompting feelings of shame and hopelessness. This might lead the client to cave in to an urge to binge (and purge). The therapist might ask, "Have you ever done this kind of eating? Do you agree with making this a target?" Usually clients nod in agreement and verbalize having similar experiences.

Decreasing Cravings, Urges, Preoccupation with Food

Clients tend to focus on or ruminate about food. This treatment assumes that such behaviors function to distract clients from distressing emotions. The therapist explains that cravings, urges, and food preoccupations are ineffective means of coping with emotions. Over time, these unattended cravings, urges, and food preoccupations can build in intensity and lead to binge eating (and purging): "Do you think this applies to you? Does it make sense to decrease that behavior? Do you agree to target it?" Clients usually respond that they are greatly troubled by cravings, urges, and preoccupations with food. Says Meredith, age 32, "I feel that certain foods, like chocolate, call out my name! It would be great to learn how to turn that off!"

Decreasing Capitulating

Capitulating is the state of mind that involves giving up or surrendering to food and eating. As the therapist explains:

> "Capitulating may seem like a passive behavior, but it is an active decision to close off your options to not binge eat [and purge]. The fact is that you always have a *choice* to binge eat [and purge] or not to. When capitulating, you are *deciding* to shut down, give up, and pull the covers over your head. Does decreasing capitulating make sense to you? Do you agree to target that behavior?"

Simon, age 42, expresses his experience with capitulating: "I end up saying 'Screw it! I'm tired of battling this!' And then I get off the highway, go to McDonald's, and end up eating four cheeseburgers in my car."

Decreasing Apparently Irrelevant Behaviors

An apparently irrelevant behavior (AIB) is a behavior that, upon first glance, does not seem relevant to binge eating (and purging) yet actually is an important component in the behavior chain leading to a binge (and purge). "This is when you tell yourself that your behavior does not matter, but deep down, you know it is setting you up." For example, Janet, a 52-year-old divorced mother, describes a typical AIB as bringing home leftover food from the office "for my son," despite the fact that she will most likely be the one to consume it. Another typical example would be buying dessert "for company" if the client is convincing him- or herself that it will be eaten by others while knowing from experience that she will likely eat it herself. Another AIB, typical of many overweight binge eaters, is avoiding the scale. By not weighing themselves, clients deprive themselves of important feedback regarding the consequences of their eating behaviors—making it easier to pretend that the binge-eating behaviors do not "really matter *that* much."

Increasing Skillful Emotion Regulation Behaviors[2]

The therapist explains that to help clients stop bingeing and take control over their eating behaviors, treatment will involve teaching adaptive emotion regulation behaviors. These skills are taught over three modules.[3]

MINDFULNESS SKILLS

Mindfulness skills facilitate the client's nonjudgmental observation, description, and experience of the current moment without having to do something to escape from it. "The basic concepts in this module are awareness and being in the present moment. Mindfulness skills can help you become more aware of your urges to binge [and purge], can help you reduce your self-judging, and can be used to replace binge eating, mindless eating, and other problem behaviors."

EMOTION REGULATION SKILLS

The skills taught in this module help the client more adaptively manage his or her emotions and break the link between emotions and problematic behaviors. The therapist elaborates:

> "The emotion of sadness, for instance, may be linked to certain behaviors, such as withdrawing and binge eating. The emotion regulation skills will teach you to experience such emotions—getting through them instead of avoiding them. Other skills involve acting in ways that are 'opposite' to your current emotion, such as becoming active rather than withdrawing. Also, even though turning to food ultimately makes you feel worse, it may also feel like your only source of pleasure. The emotion regulation skills teach ways to increase your positive emotions in healthy, enduring ways that will not backfire as binge eating does. Do these skills seem relevant to you? Do you agree to learning them?"

Typically, clients are emphatic in their agreement that these skills, especially, are relevant. Though not always (see the section on troubleshooting later in the chapter), clients usually are able to identify the link between feeling overwhelmed by their emotions (both positive and negative) and turning to food, though they are at a loss as to how to cope otherwise. The idea of specific emotion regulation skills often provides hope that through treatment they will have new and more effective ways to respond to their emotions.

---

[2]The goal of increasing skillful emotion regulation behaviors broadly refers to increasing all the adaptive skills taught (e.g., Mindfulness skills, Emotion Regulation skills, and Distress Tolerance skills)—not only those taught in the Emotion Regulation module.

[3]The adapted treatment described in this book involved teaching three skills modules, not the four of standard DBT (see also Introduction). The Interpersonal Effectiveness module was omitted due to time constraints and to limit theoretical overlap with IPT. Interpersonal issues are highly relevant with eating-disordered patients, and clinicians who wish to teach this module can find justification from a clinical standpoint. At this point, however, the inclusion of the Interpersonal Effectiveness module in this adapted treatment has not been the subject of empirical testing.

DISTRESS TOLERANCE SKILLS

These skills teach the client different ways to tolerate discomfort and distress when nothing can be done to change the situation in that moment. Distress tolerance skills include acceptance skills and skills for surviving crises.

"Not making things worse by turning to food during difficult times is an essential skill. This may mean sitting through painful emotions and urges to escape pain by observing your breath instead of turning to food. Or, in situations in which you feel emotionally overwhelmed, it may involve strategies such as taking a break or self-soothing. Does learning the skills in this module seem important to you? Do you agree to learn and practice them so that you can bear pain more skillfully instead of making matters worse with binge eating?"

Simon, who tends to binge on fast food, is typical when he says, "I hate pain! Food makes me feel better in the moment. You have your work cut out for you in teaching me something else! But if you can, more power to you! I'll give them a try."

Therapists should make it clear that the client is being asked to commit to learning and practicing *all* the skills taught during the treatment. The therapist may point out how, ultimately, of course, it is the client's choice as to which skills to continue using once treatment ends. "But you have to have be able to learn and practice all the skills in order to find out which will work best."

Following the Path to Mindful Eating

Summarizing the handout, the therapist introduces the client to research showing that *not* binge eating leads to weight loss or weight stabilization. Specifically, when abstinent from binge eating, clients with BED are more likely to lose weight, and clients with BN typically stabilize their weight (i.e., stopping purging and other compensatory behaviors does not lead to the weight gain often feared). In addition, the therapist points out (discussed in greater detail in the section on weight loss later in the chapter) that the benefits to stopping binge eating should improve the client's mood, self-esteem, and quality of life. That is, ultimately, why the client has come for treatment.

Orienting the Client to General Treatment Issues

The therapist orients the client to the general goals of treatment by saying something such as "Treatment focuses on helping you to acquire, strengthen, and apply adaptive emotion regulation behaviors to eliminate your need to rely on bingeing." Treatment is structured, with each session having a specific agenda. The client will likely find this approach quite different from others tried in the past, especially the client who has participated in "support" or "process" groups. As the therapist describes, therapy is not intended to explore the client's childhood experiences in depth nor to cover all aspects of the client's current life. In this treatment, therapist and client concentrate on issues that relate to the client's problem eating behavior. Clients typically do not raise concerns regarding the therapeutic focus. Indeed, many clients have had past treatment exploring their early childhood traumatic experiences and have noted that, although such treatment was quite helpful in many respects, it did not impact their binge-eating behaviors.

Coming Late to Sessions

Coming late to sessions is disruptive to the course of treatment. If the client knows he or she will be late, he or she should call the therapists beforehand. If the therapists have not received a prior message and the client is not present, one of the cotherapists may call to check in. As the therapist explains, doing so allows the therapist the opportunity to encourage a client who is experiencing strong urges to engage in behavior that might interfere with the therapy to use skills she or he has learned. The phone call to check in also helps allay the anxiety of group members about the whereabouts of any missing group members. Discussing lateness emphasizes the seriousness of this type of therapy-interfering behavior. In addition, the therapist needs to inform the individual client and the entire group that a persistent pattern of lateness or any other behaviors felt to be disruptive to treatment will be explored with the client.

The Therapist's Need to Interrupt

The therapist informs clients entering group treatment that to ensure that each individual has time to speak, the therapist may occasionally interrupt. Clients can expect this behavior and are requested not to take it personally.

Weight Loss

As noted, overweight clients entering treatment tend to be quite concerned about weight loss. The therapist validates the client's concerns as quite understandable. The therapist might add that he or she, too, worries about the client's weight, as the excess pounds reflect an overuse of food to numb or avoid emotions. However, the therapist makes clear that this treatment was not designed as a primary weight loss program; diet, nutrition, and meal plans are not its focus.

However, as previously addressed in the Goals of Treatment handout, clients who stop binge eating (and purging) and use adaptive skills to regulate emotions typically experience weight loss and/or weight stabilization. Specifically, the therapist may inform the client that during past trials of DBT for BED, clients lost an average of 4 pounds over the course of treatment (Telch, Agras, & Linehan, 2001). Clients who had maintained their abstinence from binge eating by 6 months following treatment lost an additional 7 pounds compared with those who relapsed, who lost 1½ pounds (Safer, Lively, Telch, & Agras, 2002).

Depending on the level of the client's concern regarding the treatment's lack of focus on weight loss or prescription of specific diet plans, the therapist might offer a more detailed rationale. Research with clients with BED has shown that many do initially respond well to the structure of being placed on a diet and tend to reduce their binge-eating behaviors. However, maintaining weight loss is difficult for many individuals, and those with BED are even more at risk of regaining lost weight (e.g., being a "yo-yo" dieter). The fact that the client is presenting for treatment exemplifies that diets are not a cure. If this treatment were to place the client on a diet, he or she might, indeed, do well. However, by virtue of not having altered the fundamental dysfunctional pattern of binge eating in response to emotional distress, the client would be at increased risk to regain that weight and feel even more defeated. Instead, it is hoped that this treatment's focus on stopping binge eating will ultimately place the client in a much better position not only to eventually diet but also to be able to maintain his or her hard-won weight loss results.

In addition, the process of dieting itself is stressful and time-consuming. Shopping for low-calorie foods, preparing meals, exercising—all necessitate effort and dedication. Although the therapist agrees that reaching a healthy weight is important, he or she wants to be realistic about what the client can achieve over the time period of treatment.

For therapists not engaged in a research study, the decision to include a weight loss component or to refer a client to a weight loss program (particularly after treatment has commenced and binge eating has improved but is not affecting weight) could be made on a case-by-case basis. Chapter 9, on future directions for research, includes a discussion of applying DBT when weight loss is a focus.

Weights of Group Members

Clients commencing group treatment occasionally express concern about how much other members will weigh. The therapist stresses that participants are of all weights and sizes. She or he can then go on to explain that all group members share a problem with an eating disorder and use food to cope with upsetting emotions.

Does the Therapist Have an Eating Disorder?

Many therapists working with clients with eating disorders encounter this question. In our experience, no clear guidelines exist as how to best respond or, indeed, whether there is an optimal answer. The therapist might express this situation to the client by saying:

> "Well, as I see it, there is not a satisfying way to answer your question. Let me show you why. If I tell you that I don't have an eating disorder, you might worry that I couldn't possibly understand your difficulties with eating enough to help you and that I would judge you. But if I said that I did have an eating disorder, you might worry that I wouldn't be able to be of help to you because I had exactly the same problem."

Or the therapist might respond: "Almost everyone in our culture has used food to cope with emotions—eating when we weren't physically hungry but felt anxious or bored. I'm hoping my not having an eating disorder won't interfere with your experience in treatment."

In a similar vein, if the client appears uncomfortable and comments about the therapist's weight (e.g., "You're so thin"), the therapist might observe that the client seems to be comparing him- or herself to the therapist and making a judgment that could interfere with the client's ability to successfully make use of this treatment opportunity. The therapist might add that he or she sincerely hopes the client will give the treatment a try despite experiencing discomfort and that during treatment, he or she will be taught skills to help cope with these types of judgments.

Patient and Therapist Treatment Agreements

The therapist hands the client a copy of the Group Member Treatment Agreements (Appendix 3.3) or Individual Client Treatment Agreements (Appendix 3.4). Each item is discussed to ensure that the client understands its rationale and to allow for questions. These agreements will be reviewed in the introductory sessions, and therefore a formal agreement is not sought during the pretreatment session. Instead, the therapist asks the client to take the form home to read and think over before bringing it back at the first session.

The therapist discusses the Therapist Treatment Agreements (Appendix 3.5) in a similar manner. These are also reviewed in Session 1.

Ending the Pretreatment Interview

Inquire whether clients have any questions that have not been answered or issues they would like to raise. Then end the interview by expressing enjoyment over having met the client and by communicating enthusiasm for working together beginning with the first session—using the opportunity to remind the client of the specific date, place, and time.

INTRODUCTORY SESSIONS

This section contains the material presented in the introductory sessions. In our 20-session research trials, this material is covered during Sessions 1 and 2. Depending on the number of sessions available and other potential factors, the therapist might proceed more slowly. Of overriding importance is the use of these introductory sessions—which complete the pretreatment stage of DBT for BED or BN—to establish the foundation for the remainder of treatment.

Sessions are described for therapists leading treatment in a group format unless otherwise noted. These descriptions can be straightforwardly modified for the therapist conducting treatment with an individual client.

In our groups, each client receives a three-ring notebook or binder. Hole-punched handouts, distributed at each session, are to be stored in this binder, which clients are instructed to bring with them to each session. We recommend that clients keep the binder readily accessible. Not only might the sight of the binder remind clients of their participation and commitment to treatment, but having it close at hand also allows them to review the content of newly taught skills and facilitates their keeping track of the work sheets by storing them in one place.

Introductions

The therapists begin by welcoming the clients to the treatment program and expressing enthusiasm about embarking on this experience together. During the pretreatment interview, each client entering group treatment will have met at least one of the two cotherapists but may not have not met the other. Each cotherapist should briefly introduce himself or herself by name, describe his or her background, and, as relevant, mention his or her position in the research project or clinic.

Therapists then ask clients to take 1–2 minutes to introduce themselves by first name and give any personal information they may wish to share (e.g., interests/hobbies, occupation, whether they have children and/or a spouse). Clients may also wish to comment on their hopes for entering treatment.

Commitment to Abstinence from Binge Eating (and Purging)

The next strategies are crucial. The therapists' goal is to build a groundswell of excitement in order to motivate clients and help them take the step to commit to abstinence from binge eating (and purging). Therapists should convey the message that abstinence from problem eating behaviors is absolutely essential if clients are to have a high quality of life. In addition, therapists should express the firm belief that this goal can be accomplished. Therapists are aiming, by the conclusion of this discussion, to have elicited a verbal commitment from each group member to stop binge eating (and purging).

The commitment strategies in DBT for BED or BN are the same as those in standard DBT (Linehan, 1993a; i.e., Evaluating Pros and Cons, Playing the Devil's Advocate, Foot in the Door, Door in the Face, Connecting Present Commitments to Prior Commitments, Highlighting Freedom to Choose in the Absence of Alternatives, and Cheerleading). Defined briefly in Chapter 2, these are described in more detail as particularly relevant. As noted, just as in standard DBT, motivation is *not* viewed as an internal state or intrinsic quality of the client. Instead, therapists understand the necessary role of situational variables that, when present, increase the likelihood that clients will exhibit a desired behavior (i.e., be "motivated"). Therapists also keep in mind that eliciting commitment and agreement from a client is an ongoing task, requiring therapists to constantly gauge the client's current level of commitment and to return to the motivation and commitment strategies as the client's commitment waxes and wanes.

Evaluating Pros and Cons is recommended as an initial technique to "sell" the commitment to abstinence from binge eating (and purging). Therapists might begin by stating:

> "It's so good to have you all finally here! We assume that you are in this room because you want to gain control over your eating behavior and stop binge eating [and purging]. We're also assuming that you want to have a full and satisfying quality of life, one in which you enjoy your relationships, experience a sense of mastery, and feel very good about yourselves most of the time. Binge eating [and purging] is a problem because it interferes with feeling good about

yourself and having the high quality of life you desire, right? Yet there are reasons why you turn to food. It has benefits. So let's begin by making an honest list of the pros and cons of continuing to be a binge eater [and purger]. The point isn't to stack the deck for one position or the other but to take the time to really look hard at the advantages and disadvantages for you of continuing this behavior. We'll start with the pros. What is the pull to remain a binger [and purger]? There must be advantages."

One cotherapist elicits the "pros" from group members, while the other writes these on a white board or large piece of paper. (Note: If conducting treatment within an individual format, the therapist may list the pros on a piece of paper.) After eliciting the pros of binge eating (and purging), therapists inquire about the cons: "What are the serious disadvantages to remaining a binge eater [and purger]? What types of things brought you into treatment?" Again, one therapist elicits these and the other writes them down. Once the lists are created, therapists should use the strategy *Playing the Devil's Advocate* to help solidify the motivation:

"Those pros look pretty darn compelling! We're not sure we'd be able to find a way to say to ourselves that we would work like heck to give up bingeing [and purging]. *Convince us*—why can't you continue to binge eat [and purge] and still lead a highly satisfying life? Now, when we refer to this quality of life, we're not talking about a life in which you're simply existing or 'getting through' and trying to minimize pain. We're talking about feeling fully alive, living up to your potential, having the best life that you're capable of."

When Playing Devil's Advocate, therapists draw group members into arguing the position that it is imperative for them to stop binge eating (and purging) in order to live the quality of life clients most desire. The therapists remain skeptical, continuing to wonder aloud whether clients might indeed be able to continue binge eating (and purging) while simultaneously living a fully satisfying life. The key to this strategy's success is polarizing the argument by describing clearly and reiterating as needed what is meant by a high quality of life. If this is done, most clients readily argue that their binge eating (and purging) is destroying any possibility of their having a high quality of life.

When the therapists are convinced that the group is strongly in agreement, they might summarize:

"Based on what we have heard from you, we're convinced that there is absolutely no other choice than to stop binge eating [and purging] and to get control over any other problem eating behaviors. So, let's face that reality and put it on the table before we move ahead. Binge eating [and purging] is over. Whenever you had your last binge [and/or purge], that was it—the last one. You simply can't have the life you want and continue this kind of eating. If you stop all these problem eating behaviors, you have a shot at the life you want to lead. But if you continue, you simply don't have a chance. So the only choice you've got is to stop binge eating [and purging]. Are we truly agreed?"

Getting Verbal Commitment to Abstinence from Binge Eating and/or Purging

The next step is obtaining each client's verbal commitment to abstinence. The therapists explain this request as follows:

> "One thing we believe would be helpful, according to our model, is for you to make a commitment to stop binge eating [and purging]. The reason we say this is that we know from the research that there is a power to making a commitment that isn't there when you simply say: 'I'll try.' People who make a *commitment* to do something are more likely to follow through. So we're asking you to make a verbal commitment, to look deeply within yourselves and make a decision to give up binge eating [and purging] as an ineffective way of coping with emotional distress."

Therapists then ask clients to take a moment to think over the discussion that just took place, reminding them that it was they who convinced the therapists about the incompatibility of binge eating (and purging) and living a high-quality life: "This is not something we are telling you, this is something you know in a deep way, based on your own experiences. Stay in touch with the high cost of binge eating [and purging] and find a way to make a deep commitment to yourself and to the treatment to give up this behavior."

Therapists then address each client: "Can you say, 'I commit to stop binge eating [and purging]'?" Once all clients have made the commitment, take a 5- to 10-minute break between the first and second hours of the group session.

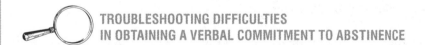 TROUBLESHOOTING DIFFICULTIES
IN OBTAINING A VERBAL COMMITMENT TO ABSTINENCE

In our groups, clients have differing reactions to being asked to make a verbal commitment to binge abstinence. Most tend to find it fairly straightforward, but some clients express a number of concerns and negative emotions (e.g., anxiety, anger). The observed discomfort and distress often is shared by therapists, who likely experience a pull to soften or lessen the commitment that is asked for. Given the research to date on this treatment's effectiveness is based on the protocol described in this book, we strongly recommend that therapists push for the highest level of commitment from clients that can be obtained. The following approaches should prove useful.

• *Example 1*: "I won't be able to keep the commitment. It's impossible. So I can't make this commitment."

• *Potential therapist reply*: "Would it literally be impossible to keep the commitment? I mean, it would likely be very, very difficult and scary—but are you saying that you think there is no way for you to physically survive unless you continue binge eating [and purging] ?" If the client concedes that it actually would be possible to survive while abstaining, therapists might add: "So, it sounds like you agree it might actually be possible to stop bingeing [and purging], but you are very certain that you would fail in the attempt. Therefore it feels easier to tell yourself that stopping binge eating [and purging] is impossible. Because if you were to try your best but fail, you would have to feel awful about yourself not only for having binged [and/or purged] but also for failing in your attempt to stop. I can understand that kind of thinking. Yet we know from research on commitments that when people don't make a full commitment—when, right from the outset they say there's no hope—the likelihood of success is lower."

Other optional therapist replies include: *"Are you worried about binge eating [and purging] in this moment, or are you worried about the future?"* Reassure the client that therapists are not talking about anything but this one moment, reminding them that, after all, life is only made up of a continuous set of present moments. "Can you make a commitment to try your absolute hardest to never ever binge [and purge] again in this one moment, right now?" (Foot-in-the-Door Technique; Linehan, 1993a, pp. 288–289). If the client replies that he or she can make a commitment for this one moment, therapists can ask for a moment more, and so on.

- *Example 2*: "Okay. I'll commit to trying."
- *Potential therapist reply*: "We really appreciate your willingness to give this a shot. But we also know from research, as well as from our experience with this treatment, that when people say they'll 'try,' they are leaving the door open, even just a crack, for turning to binge eating when it gets really hard. In a sense 'trying' is saying 75% of me will be on board, but if it gets really bad, I'm going to go back to binge eating. It's actually in that 25% of the time that reminding yourself of your absolute commitment to *no* binge eating will make it much more likely that you will make it through without food. So let's really step back and try to understand what is making it hard for you to 100% commit."

(Note: If the client continues to insist on "trying" as being the best he or she can do, the therapist may decide that this response can be shaped over time. Until that point, the therapist—to be adherent to this treatment—must hold firm to the idea that binge eating *can* be stopped and that a 100% commitment can be made, even if the commitment has to be made and renewed one moment at a time. Indeed, as discussed, clients can be reminded that life is only a series of moments.)

- *Example 3*: "I can't commit because it would be a setup to binge [and purge]."
- *Potential therapist reply*: "You're worried about committing—you think that if you do, you're setting yourself up. You'd commit here and then go straight out to binge [and purge] after the group is over?" We have found it helpful to ask, "Is it impossible to have a goal and at the same time not meet it? Does it make it wrong to have the goal?"

(Note: This response illustrates the concept of dialectical abstinence, which is formally introduced during the next session.)

- *Example 4*: "This doesn't feel right. I feel like I'm being forced to make this commitment."

- *Potential therapist reply*: "I'm so glad you spoke up! I'm sure others feel this way. We cannot be clear enough that only you can decide whether or not you want to make this commitment. It is absolutely your life and your choice. The benefits of binge eating [and purging] may truly be greater for you than the negative consequences. If so, it would make sense that you wouldn't be willing to commit to giving them up. If need be, you're willing to live with the consequences—the health problems, the lowered self-esteem, not having the high quality of life we talked about." Therapists stay silent long enough for the client to digest this (highlighting freedom to choose and absence of alternatives; Linehan 1993a, pp. 289–290).

- *Example 5*: "Life would *not* be so bad if I could just cut down on my binge eating [and purging]—if I could just do it less often or binge on vegetables."

- *Potential therapist reply*: "Well, you're right that it would definitely be a big improvement if you binged [and/or purged] less often. But my understanding of a high-quality life is that in order to feel fully alive, fully responsive to each moment that life gives you, it's not possible to simultaneously avoid life or numb yourself with food. Choosing to do something so destructive to yourself, can you at the same time live to your full potential?" Again, therapists stay silent and do not push.

- *Example 6*: "I can't imagine a life without binge eating [and purging]. I'm too scared to make the commitment."

- *Potential therapist reply*: "Is it hard for you to imagine what a high quality of life looks like, so you aren't sure what you are striving for?" Many people with BED or BN become so accustomed to a lowered quality of life that they begin to feel as if nothing more is possible. Therapists can gently point out that they are asking the client to envision having a life that may indeed seem impossible, one that may feel as if it is too much for the client to want for him- or herself: "It *is* scary, but I think you can do it. I think you can let yourself want your life to be that good."

Pros or Cons of Binge Eating

This next skill involves summarizing the pros-and-cons discussion that took place prior to the verbal commitment. To strengthen the commitment that has just been made and to remind clients of their personal reasons for making and upholding the commitment to stop binge eating, therapists distribute 3″ × 5″ index cards. They instruct clients to list their five worst consequences of binge eating (and purging) on one side. On the other, clients should list the five most positive consequences of not binge eating (and purging). Clients may find it helpful to look at the white board pros and cons generated from the group discussion to stimulate their thinking.

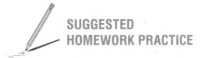

SUGGESTED
HOMEWORK PRACTICE

1. Therapists instruct clients to practice the skill of committing to binge (and purge) abstinence by slowing down, taking a few deep breaths, and finding a soft place for their eyes to focus. Clients should then practice recommitting in their "heart of hearts" to no more binge eating (and purging). Therapists might add:

"Try to stay with that feeling, that firm commitment, and the strength and clarity that accompanies it."

   2. Therapists suggest that when clients experience even the slightest thought or urge to binge (and purge), they should bring to mind the promise they made to themselves, as well as imagining the therapists and the entire group saying, "We are all rock solid behind you in this."

   3. Therapists instruct clients to review their 3" × 5" cards with the pros and cons at least once a day, as well as at any time they experience urges to binge (and purge). Therapists might suggest that clients make multiple copies of these cards to allow easy and quick reference, keeping the cards in readily accessible locations such as one's wallet or purse.

Orientation to Treatment

Treatment Model, Assumptions, and Rationale

Therapists begin this next section by congratulating clients on having been able to make, for themselves, the commitment to strive for a higher quality of life by stopping binge eating. At this point, as therapists explain, greater detail will be given about the treatment, including its underlying assumptions and the model, both of which were briefly introduced in the pretreatment interview.

   Present the essential treatment model, perhaps by saying:

"This is how we understand binge eating [and purging]. First, there is a trigger or prompting event. We don't believe binge eating [and purging] occurs for no reason, even though sometimes the trigger may not be easy to pinpoint. Similarly, we don't think binge eating is a habit that serves no purpose nor an addiction you have no control over. We believe it is something that you have learned to do and can unlearn. So, first, something happens. We refer to this as a prompting event."

To help clients generate ideas about possible prompting events for them, the therapist may find it useful to offer some illustrations: "For example, one prompting event might be looking at your closet in the morning and telling yourself that you have nothing that fits. It could also be experiencing your clothes as tight during the day." For Marie, a college student, typical prompting events for binges were having exams to study for or receiving a grade lower than she had hoped for. For Sarah, the mother of two younger children, not having her husband home at night was a frequent trigger.

"The prompting event does not have to be a major event—it is just an event, such as being alone in the house, that sets off an emotion that makes you uncomfortable. And according to our model, this uncomfortable emotion is something you want to go away or at least lessen in either duration or intensity or both. Even positive emotions like joy can feel uncomfortable if you don't know how to manage them. And our assumption is that people with binge eating [and purging] problems have an underdeveloped, inadequate emotion regulation system. This includes deficits in monitoring, evaluating, modifying, and accepting emotional experiencing. You haven't acquired the skills to regulate your emotions.

"Food 'solves' this problem, so to speak. Temporarily it provides a way of lessening your emotional experience by soothing you, helping you numb out, taking your attention, and so forth. But the relief gained, as you know, is only temporary. Using food doesn't teach you effective ways of coping with your emotional distress and therefore doesn't solve the underlying deficit. The next time an uncomfortable feeling comes up, the link you've made between emotional upset and eating is that much stronger.

"We think the problem *is not* the emotion you experience, the emotion that was triggered. In our view, the problem is the behavior you've learned to use to cope with your emotions. In the long run, this behavior seriously lowers the quality of your life, leading to more distress. It does not work to achieve the desired effect of helping you feel better. It may provide a temporary distraction, but eventually it causes more misery. It also may inhibit more adaptive emotional behaviors, such as asking for help. Numbing emotions with food leads to a reduced chance of receiving validation, help, support, and the possibility of change. It interferes with behaviors that may lead to true improvements in your life.

"We want to help you break the link between having uncomfortable emotions and turning to food to cope. We will teach you more skillful ways of regulating your emotions so you can stop binge eating [and purging] and replace the dysfunctional behaviors. These skills for gaining emotional control may reduce emotional experiencing before the emotion starts in the first place, or they may modify the behavioral expression of an emotion that has already been experienced. At this point, we're not sure whether you just don't have the skills in your repertoire to act differently or whether the maladaptive eating is so overlearned that it crowds out skilled behaviors that you do have. We are assuming that even if you have some of these skills, you can still benefit from a refresher to strengthen their use; you can also acquire new skills and practice the skillful behaviors."

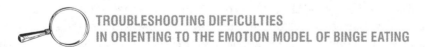

TROUBLESHOOTING DIFFICULTIES IN ORIENTING TO THE EMOTION MODEL OF BINGE EATING

- *Example*: "I don't think I have any emotions before I binge. I don't notice any—just the urge to binge."

- *Potential therapist reply*: "We believe that people are always experiencing emotions. But because you have learned to turn to food so quickly to deal with emotions, you may not even be aware of them. Perhaps you have a glimmer of discomfort but all you're aware of is 'That dessert looks awfully good.' We will help you in this program get more skillful at observing and describing your emotions."

The Biosocial Model

This section involves giving clients background into the development of what this model assumes is the primary and central problem in clients with disordered eating—an underdeveloped, inadequate emotion regulation system with deficits in monitoring, evaluating, modifying, and accepting their emotional experiencing (see also related material in Chapter 2). In other words, clients with binge eating (and purging) difficulties often feel depressed, angry, anxious, and out of control of their emotions. The inability to regulate emotion interferes with achieving and maintaining a positive self-view and leads to low self-esteem. This, in turn, may make them more emotionally vulnerable. Deficits in emotion regulation are believed to stem from a variety of factors.

One assumption that makes it harder for clients with binge eating (and purging) problems to cope with their emotions is that they have a biologically based increased emotional sensitivity compared with other individuals. It may not hold true for all clients, yet, in our experience, individuals with BED and BN often agree with this information and describe having been told throughout their lives that they are "too sensitive."

 DISCUSSION POINT:
"Have you been told that you're too sensitive, too 'thin skinned'?"

A second assumption is that when clients with eating disorders do react, they tend to have very strong impulses to act on their emotions and strong reactions to their emotional experience, such as a sense that their hearts are pounding harder and so forth. This emotional sensitivity, combined with a deficit in the ability to adaptively regulate emotions, creates a very difficult situation. Bingeing and purging are mood-dependent behaviors, and when feelings and urges to act on those emotions arise, it is very hard to refrain from engaging in that behavior. This treatment teaches skills to help clients gain control of emotions and behaviors so that the two are not so tightly linked. It helps clients learn to tolerate strong feelings without having to *do* something to stop them.

The Invalidating Environment

Another assumption of this model is that disordered eating behaviors develop through an interaction between the client's biologically based emotional sensitivity and a certain set of conditions, called the *invalidating environment*. In the invalidating environment, emotions were not given time to be noticed or talked about. On those occasions when they were noticed, they were not labeled accurately or taken to be important. This set of circumstances would naturally cause individuals to have difficulty in knowing and being able to label their feelings, in trusting their own emotions as valid interpretations of what is taking place, and in adaptively regulating their emotional arousal and reactions. It would be hard to tolerate distress. And, indeed, if individuals were punished for expressing their emotions, over time they would have learned to control and dampen down their emotions—eventually deciding not to show them or feel them. Instead, they would learn to push away their emotional experiences, thereby self-invalidating their feelings. Over time, they may have learned that food helps them to do this quite well.

We have found the following teaching illustration helpful for demonstrating to clients what we mean by the invalidating environment.

Illustrating the Invalidating Environment

Suggest that clients imagine a situation in which a small child goes to a carnival and wins a goldfish. Furthermore, they should picture a child who is emotionally sensitive in the ways that were just described. Compared with other children, this child has more powerful emotional reactions. When the child wins the goldfish, for example, he or she is absolutely overcome with joy—bouncing the bag up and down, looking at the fish repeatedly, poking at it through the bag, and so forth. The child is clearly terrifically excited and caught up in that excitement. Clients are then asked to imagine that the following day the goldfish dies. The child is devastated and cries and cries—unable to stop sobbing about his or her disappointment and desire for the goldfish to come back. Therapists explain that in the invalidating environment, the caregivers—for whatever reason—cannot tolerate their child's intense experience and expression of emotion. Perhaps the caregivers had grown up in invalidating environments themselves or are depressed. In any case, the caregivers feel the need to try to shut down the child's emotions. In this scenario, the caregivers unceremoniously flush the fish down the toilet, saying: "Shut up! Why are you crying? You only had that goldfish for a day! If you don't stop crying, I'll give you something to cry about!" Therapists highlight how the child's inner experience is not validated in this environment. With repeated episodes such as this (not just a few), the child would learn not to trust his or her emotions. The child would likely believe that something is wrong with him or her for feeling as he or she does.

Therapists might also find it useful to offer another example, saying something such as:

> "Thirst is an inner experience most people have no difficulty recognizing. But imagine that you were raised in a household where that experience was invalidated because for some reason it was difficult for your caregivers to respond to. After years of being told, 'You're not thirsty, you just had a drink of water,' how do you feel you would react? Most likely, you would have difficulty knowing your internal experience of thirst or how to handle it. That is what we're saying it is like when your emotions are invalidated."

According to the model, another characteristic of the invalidating environment is that every once in a while the child's extreme emotional display may be reinforced. For example, the caregiver might react with sympathy when the child seems especially overcome with emotion. This teaches the child to escalate the emotional expression the next time, such as a child who is reinforced with candy when his or her cries and tears become exceptionally strong. Therapists explain that when rewards are given on an intermittent basis (e.g., intermittent reinforcement), those related behaviors are particularly difficult to change. In such punishing and intermittently reinforcing environments, the child would not learn to communicate his or her emotional pain or distress effectively.

Another characteristic of the invalidating environment is that the child is told overly simplistic methods for problem solving and regulating emotions, such as "Just smile and the world will smile with you," "Just decide not to feel that way," or "Pull yourself up by your own bootstraps!" Because of oversimplifying, the child is not taught to tolerate distress or to solve the difficult and complex problems of living. Instead, he or she is likely to form unrealistic goals and to become highly distressed by failure.

Illustrating Validating Environments

Revisit the imaginary scenario with the child who wins the goldfish. Ask clients to picture the same highly emotionally sensitive child, now devastated by the death of the goldfish. Yet in this scenario the caregivers, for whatever reason, have more emotional resources. "Imagine the effect if the caregivers respond by saying, 'Oh, you're sad. It hurts to have something you love die when you didn't want it to. I can see how much you wish things were different. How about writing a poem about it? We'll have a funeral ceremony and you can read it.'" The child in this environment learns, with repeated episodes such as this, to trust his or her emotions as valid. The therapists explain that although the child would always be emotionally sensitive, he or she would be more likely to learn ways to adaptively regulate his or her emotional arousal.

◉ **DISCUSSION POINT:** *"The consequences of having an invalidating environment may include not being able to label your feelings, not trusting your emotions as valid, not being able to regulate your emotions, and having a low tolerance for distress. Basically this means not trusting your emotions about what is going on around you and judging yourself as wrong for feeling as you do. Does that seem to fit for any of you?"*

Therapists might conclude this section by saying:

"The good news is that what was learned in the past can be unlearned. Although we won't be spending our time exploring the origins of the emotional experiences you had in your childhood, we will be focusing on correcting the skill deficits that may have resulted. Indeed, this therapy is in some ways the Emotions 101 course you may have never had. Our treatment program will help you express your emotions and enable you to live your life without using food as a solution to emotional distress. We also assume that some problems can't be solved, but that it's better to live with the problem than with a destructive solution. You will learn to replace your maladaptive responses with adaptive skills for gaining emotional control."

Reviewing Goals of Treatment, Skills Training, Treatment Targets

The goals of treatment, though introduced in the pretreatment interview, are reviewed again in these introductory sessions due to their importance in providing a firm foundation for the remainder of the treatment.

We suggest handing out hole-punched copies of the handout (Appendix 3.2) Goals of Treatment, Goals of Skills Training, and Treatment Targets (as modified for the therapists' particular client population) and reviewing it in detail. For example, therapists might say:

> "Again, what is really important to you and is the reason you joined this program is that you want to stop binge eating [and purging]. So that is our overall goal. The basic premise of this treatment program is that by learning and practicing adaptive and skillful ways to cope with emotions, you will be able to use the skills to replace your maladaptive binge eating [and purging], other problem eating behaviors, and other maladaptive means you currently use to cope with your emotions."

Then review the path to mindful eating, either by discussing each point in turn or by asking clients to recall from the pretreatment interview what these behaviors entail. In either case, therapists should elicit a general commitment as to the importance of each before moving ahead.

TREATMENT-INTERFERING BEHAVIOR

As the therapist explained in the pretreatment interview, even more important than getting clients to stop problem eating is to prioritize any behavior that interferes with coming to treatment, learning the skills, or practicing them. Without fully receiving the treatment, how will anything improve? Do clients agree to work on solving any such problems if they come up?

STOPPING BINGE EATING (AND PURGING)

As discussed, and as clients have already agreed, this is a "must" to gain a higher quality of life.

The treatment then targets behaviors that are believed to set clients up to binge eat (and purge), beginning with eliminating mindless eating.

ELIMINATING MINDLESS EATING

Therapists review how this includes eating when clients are not paying attention. Have clients ever experienced having a bowl of snacks in front of them while watching television, then noticing that all the snacks are gone without recalling actually eating them all? How do they react in such situations? Often, such eating leads to a binge (and purge). Mindless eating also includes eating chaotically (e.g., throughout an evening) and never planning a meal. Though it may not feel like a loss of control, this type of eating can lead to binge eating (and purging).

DECREASING GENERAL PREOCCUPATION WITH FOOD, URGES, AND CRAVINGS

Clients with eating disorders report thinking about food a great deal of the time—finding themselves preoccupied by it and experiencing food-related urges and cravings. This program assumes that these behaviors set clients up to eventually binge eat (and purge) and therefore must be targeted. Ruminating about food, for instance, can be a way to distract oneself from upsetting emotions. Because these behaviors do not teach clients to cope effectively with their emotions, the preoccupation can lead to binge eating (and purging).

DECREASING CAPITULATING

Therapists might use this opportunity to remind clients that they always have a choice about whether or not to binge eat (and purge). Although it may feel as if they *must* do it, the reality is that individuals do *not* die if they are not able to binge (and purge). The mind-set one enters into, called capitulating, may seem passive, but it is an active process. It involves actively closing off options, deciding to give up and to surrender to eating. It is a willful shutdown. Capitulating is maladaptive behavior that sets one up to binge (and purge), and it may be a behavior that clients recognize they use more generally.

DECREASING AIBs

AIBs are behaviors that clients pretend or try to convince themselves do not set them up for binge eating (and purging) despite knowing deep down that these behaviors are risky. Examples include making the decision to go grocery shopping when feeling particularly vulnerable to urges to overeat (but rationalizing that one is "simply going to buy milk") or buying bake sale items at a fundraiser (instead of offering a donation). Ask clients to give examples from their lives.

To stop bingeing (and purging) and get control over their eating, clients will be replacing their problem eating behaviors with adaptive skills for gaining emotional control. These are taught over three modules.[4]

Mindfulness Skills. These skills increase awareness and experience of the current moment without self-consciousness or judgment. These are the core skills of the treatment program.

Emotion Regulation Skills. These skills include helping clients identify emotions, understand their function, reduce vulnerability to negative emotions, and increase positive emotions. By understanding how emotions work, clients are

---

[4]As mentioned earlier in this chapter and in the Introduction, the treatment manual described is based on using the three modules as presented. Decisions about the number of modules were based on the population studied and research issues (e.g., omitting the Interpersonal Effectiveness module to limit theoretical overlap with IPT). Interpersonal issues are highly relevant with patients who have eating disorders. Therapists may decide to add this module, but the decision to do so has not yet been the subject of empirical testing within our research protocols with patients who have BED or BN.

more able to regulate them. This may include reducing the intensity of an emotion before it gets fully going, modifying the way the emotion expresses itself once it has already started, and/or acting in ways that are "opposite" to the current emotion.

Distress Tolerance Skills. These skills include Crisis Survival skills and acceptance skills to help clients tolerate distressing emotional states in situations that cannot, in that moment, be changed.

It is expected that clients will learn and practice all the skills so that they can find out which ones ultimately will work best for them.

Therapists might reinforce the fact that abstinence from binge eating (and purging), according to research, leads to weight stabilization or weight loss (see also earlier discussion and Chapter 2). In addition, if clients stop bingeing (and purging), it is expected that their moods will improve, as should their self-esteem and overall quality of life.

Orientation to Structure of Sessions

The structure of sessions is described to give clients a sense of the format of each weekly session. Group sessions, per our research protocol, last 2 hours and include 8–12 clients. Depending on therapists' clinic settings and client populations, groups might be extended to 2½ hours. The first half (50–60 minutes in our groups) is devoted to reviewing the past week's skills practice, diary card, and chain analyses—as will be described. After a 5- to 10-minute break, the second half of the session is devoted to teaching specific skills.

Sessions carried out in an individual format last 50–60 minutes. The same session structure is maintained, with the first 25–30 minutes used to review the client's prior week of skills practice (including review of the diary card, chain analysis, etc.), followed by teaching new skills for the remainder of the session.

Especially when sessions are carried out in a group format with 10 or so clients, we find it necessary to structure the sharing to ensure that each group member has a chance to speak (see also discussion in Chapter 2). We review this structure in greater detail in subsequent sessions. The point for therapists to communicate at this juncture is that each group member is expected to share his or her practice of the skills each week during the first half of group. In groups with 10 clients, this means approximately 5 minutes per group member. Therapists emphasize that structuring this first half is needed given that this is a time-limited treatment program that focuses on skill acquisition and strengthening. Treatment is not intended, as has been noted, to cover all aspects of clients' lives or to handle all crises. Current difficulties can be discussed insofar as they relate to the skills being taught. The idea is that learning to use adaptive emotion regulation skills will ultimately enhance clients' ability to cope with all areas of their lives.

For clients to make maximal use of treatment, it is important for them to plan ahead as to what they most want to discuss. Clients have the opportunity to review their practice of the skills over the previous week (i.e., what worked out, what they would like help with) and to report from their chain analysis, a tool that analyzes the client's engagement in problem behaviors over the prior week.

Therapists remind clients of the dates of sessions scheduled during this course of treatment. Although our research trials were based on a 20-session format, the number of sessions may vary depending on differences in client settings and treatment populations.

Group Member and Therapist Treatment Agreements

The Group Member and Therapist Treatment Agreements (Appendices 3.3 and 3.5), initially discussed during the pretreatment interview, are handed out and reviewed in the introductory sessions. Therapists read each of the items on the agreement aloud, emphasizing that these agreements are essential to provide optimal conditions under which group members can receive benefit from the treatment.

As the therapists explain, *confidentiality*, or keeping information about what group members say private, is vital to create a safe environment in which group members feel free to openly discuss highly personal issues and feelings. Not forming private relationships with other group members that would interfere with the vital ability of the group to function as a whole, such as forming exclusive cliques, is also important. In turn, the therapists agree not to form private relationships with clients that would be disruptive.

Therapists underscore the expectation that group members will prioritize this experience and protect the group session time so that they can attend regularly. Absences should be only those that are truly unavoidable, such as the case of serious illness or out-of-town trips that cannot be rescheduled. It is asked that group members call the therapist (or a designated person) if they will miss a session so that the group can be informed and not worry about the absent group member. As described earlier, therapists may also call clients who are expected at group but are not present at the start of the group session. The therapist takes this opportunity to emphasize that clients are expected to complete homework each week even if the session was missed. In our research trials, group sessions were recorded, allowing missed sessions to be made up by having group members come in to watch or listen to the videotape or audiotape. This held true, as we pointed out in our research trials, for therapists as well. If a cotherapist missed a session, he or she agreed to listen to the missed session before the next group meeting. If a cotherapist has a planned absence, he or she agrees to inform the group of this ahead of time.

Review the commitment to practice the skills taught and to abstain from binge eating (and purging). In a research setting, in which completion of research assessments is required and is included in a treatment agreement, therapists explain that cooperation with such assessments is essential for evaluating the current treatment program to create therapies that are as effective as possible.

After reviewing the group agreements, the therapists might ask, "Now that you've reviewed these, do you feel you can sign them? If so, sign them and turn them in." After collecting the group agreements, the therapists should read through the therapist agreements (several of which have been referred to in the preceding discussion). In our research groups, both cotherapists sign these agreements ahead of the session so that copies can be made. Before handing them out, therapists might say: "Just as you are working very hard, we are equally committed to working very hard to help you achieve your goal of stopping binge eating [and purging]. These are our agreements. We have signed them and are giving you copies."

Introduction to the Chain Analysis

Hand out a Sample Chain Analysis and Guidelines for Filling Out a Behavioral Chain Analysis of a Problem Behavior (Appendices 3.6 and 3.7), if not already included in each client's binder. Blank copies of the chain analysis (Appendix 3.8) are handed out as well. Therapists introduce the chain analysis as an invaluable tool. Though it requires time and effort to fill out, it provides essential detail for understanding the events that lead up to binge eating (and purging). Clients will be asked to fill one out for the next session (with guidance from the sample chain and the instructions). Once they have had some experience with it, clients will have the opportunity to have more questions answered. (For further discussion of chain analysis, see pp. 61–63.)

The purpose of a behavioral analysis is to figure out what the problem (e.g., binge eating and purging) is, what triggers it, what its function is, what is interfering with the resolution of the problem, and what aids are available to help solve the problem. Many errors in treatment of eating disorders are made because the problem at hand is not fully understood and assessed.

Clients are referred to the top of the first page of the sample chain analysis, the diagram of a chain. The main point to make is that binge eating and purging, like any behavior, can be understood as being made up of a series of components or links. These links are chained together. As the therapists describe, behaviors that are well rehearsed, such as binge eating (and purging), are often experienced as occurring "lightning fast." Clients often have great difficulty describing how they got from Point A, at which they were not binge eating (and purging), to Point B, at which they were. It feels out of control and can have a "blurry" quality. The importance of using the chain analysis is to break down what seems lightning fast into an understandable sequence of events. Emphasize that binge eating and purging are *learned* behaviors and thus can be *unlearned*. The pattern linking the components together *can* be identified. Furthermore, by breaking any of the links, the chain to binge eating and purging *can* be broken.

The chain analysis worksheet asks clients to identify what exactly the problem behavior was, what the vulnerabilities were that made them more likely to engage in it, what the prompting event was that triggered things, what the specific links were, and what consequences resulted.

The first step is identifying the problem behavior. Therapists explain that clients should refer to the path to mindful eating (Appendix 3.2) and analyze the highest target behavior that occurred between sessions. It is most important to target any behavior that interferes with treatment. In other words, if clients are not practicing the skills, they should write a chain on that problem behavior. Next, binge episodes and/or purges would be targeted, followed by mindless eating, and so forth.

The chain analysis worksheet then asks clients to identify the prompting event. Therapists explain that this is something occurring in the environment that started the chain of events off. The third box on the work sheet focuses on identification of vulnerability factors. Vulnerability factors occur before the prompting event and include those factors that make the client more susceptible to the prompting event, such as internal issues (e.g., an illness, being fatigued) or external features (e.g., having no one else at home, facing tempting foods at a buffet or party).

Next, clients are asked to imagine that the problem behavior is chained to the prompting event. Therapists remind them that prompting events are external to the client. Following that, what were the links, the specific thoughts, actions, bodily sensations, or events that took place? Once these are identified, clients are to describe what followed them. After describing the links, clients are to try to think of what they could have done differently at each link to break the chain. In particular, clients are asked to identify what skills could have been used—such as referring to the 3″ × 5″ card or renewing their commitment to stop binge eating (and purging).

The last page asks clients to identify the consequences of the binge (and purge), ways to reduce their vulnerability, things they could do to prevent the prompting event from happening again, and questions about the harm that was caused. In addition, when the client feels harm has been caused by the binge eating (and purging) and experiences guilt and remorse, he or she may also consider what could be done to repair the damage to themselves and others, if applicable.[5]

The therapist should emphasize the following:

• Clients should not get "hung up" on trying to fill out the chain *perfectly* or getting it *exactly* right. The most important thing is that clients begin to actually use the chain. The sample chain and instructions for filling it out can serve as guides. Greater detail is provided in future sessions.

• Key dysfunctional links: When filling out the list of links on the second page of the chain, clients should try to focus on the key dysfunctional link(s)—the link or links (e.g., a particular thought, feeling, event, or action) that seem most associated with hooking or chaining together the prompting event (i.e., an external event or cue triggering the chain) with the problem behavior. The therapist should make clear that links may be functional or dysfunctional. It is how the client responds to the link that may bring him or her closer to or farther from the problem behavior.

• Clients will find, based on their experience with filling out chains over time, how important it is to gain increased awareness of their thoughts and feelings—something the invalidating environment discouraged.

• At times, clients will have a lot to write in their chains. At other times, less so.

---

[5]In standard DBT, repairing harm is part of the egregious-behavior protocol and is used when clients have caused harm to others (e.g., stealing). Binge-eating behaviors typically do not cause harm to others so much as to the client him- or herself and are often accompanied by excessive guilt or remorse. In such instances, correction and overcorrection may be helpful, and thus they are included in the standard form for the chain analysis used in this treatment.

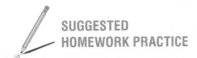

**SUGGESTED
HOMEWORK PRACTICE**

Therapists instruct clients to fill out at least one chain analysis between sessions so as to gain adequate practice with this essential tool. Clients may, of course, wish to fill out additional chains.

Introduction to Diary Cards

If they are not already included in the client's binder, the therapists hand out copies of the Diary Card and Instructions for Filling Out a Diary Card (Appendices 3.9 and 3.10) to each group member. The diary card's primary purpose is to remind clients to practice the skills during the week and to give them a place to record that practice. It is also a space in which to keep track of targeted behaviors (e.g., binge eating [and purging] and other behaviors on the path to mindful eating). Clients are also asked to record their experience of different emotions (e.g., anger, sadness, fear, happiness) each day and to notice patterns between those emotions and the use of targeted behaviors. (Note: For clients with BED, modify the Diary Card by omitting the "purge" columns and subdividing binge episodes into large ["objective"] and small ["subjective"] as described in Appendix 3.10. See also Wisniewski et al. [2007, p. 217].)

In addition, as emphasized, this treatment puts at the very top of the treatment hierarchy any behaviors that interfere with therapy. Therapists explain that, therefore, clients are asked to rate their urges to quit therapy—both before and after sessions—on the diary card. The therapists might mention that they will be paying special attention to that rating.

In our research protocols, clients are asked to weigh themselves once a week and record that weight on the diary card. Not weighing, as described, can be an AIB for many clients. If clients report that weighing themselves has been a trigger to binge eating (and purging) in the past, we suggest that they weigh themselves right before a session. It is vital for clients not to avoid triggers, and this would allow them to get support from the group for using skills to help tolerate the emotions experienced after stepping on the scale.

The reverse side of the diary card lists the adaptive emotion regulation skills in the order taught in our research protocols. Clients are asked to circle the skill on the day that they practiced it.

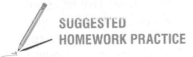

**SUGGESTED
HOMEWORK PRACTICE**

Therapists recommend that clients fill out their diary cards at least once a day. These cards are reviewed at the beginning of each session.

(Note: As cannot be overemphasized, without practice, clients will not be successful at changing a long-standing behavior such as binge eating and purging. Ideally, clients will keep their diary cards with them during the day to facilitate accurate records of skills practiced and use of the targeted behaviors. It is helpful to review the card at the end of the day to make sure that all the skills practiced and all targeted behaviors were recorded. For additional directions on filling out the diary card, clients can refer to Instructions for Filling Out a Diary Card [Appendix 3.10].)

Structuring the Client's First Report of Skills Practice

As brought up in the introduction and Chapter 2, one of the distinctive features of this adapted treatment as opposed to standard DBT is that the functions of individual therapy and group skills training are brought together. Specifically, enhancing motivation (typically done in individual psychotherapy) and acquiring/ strengthening new skills (typically occurring within a skills training context) are separated in standard DBT, whereas in DBT as adapted for binge eating (and purging), these functions are combined into one session.

For therapists using a group format for treatment, the most challenging element of therapy involves conducting this first half of the treatment session, beginning with Session 2. Following are some of the ideas we have found helpful:

- On a white board (or handout), write general guidelines about how therapists would like clients to report on their skills practice during their allotted time (e.g., 5 minutes). In our groups, we suggest that clients follow the guidelines outlined in Appendix 3.11.
- Therapists may wish to remind clients (particularly during the early sessions) of the skills taught so far by writing them on the board as well.
- Therapists can emphasize that, because each client has a limited period of time, the therapists really hope clients will use it maximally.

Therapists might make the following points:

- "We'd like to start out with your letting us know whether you had a binge episode [and purge] or not during the prior week, followed by answering questions regarding your skill practice. This week, for example, the skills from our first session that you were to have practiced were the commitment, the 3″ × 5″ card, and filling out the diary card itself. If you had a question or difficulty with the homework, this would be the place to bring that up so we can help you."
- "If you didn't practice the skills or did not fill out a diary card or chain analysis, we would like to understand with you what got in the way. This is important because, as you'll remember from the goals of treatment, our top goal—even before stopping binge eating [and purging]—is to not engage in therapy-interfering behavior. If you could do this on your own, you would have! In our experience, clients who successfully used this program to stop binge eating [and purging] did their homework and attended sessions."
- "After reporting on your diary card and your practice of skills, we'd like you to report on your chain analysis. Please use the chain analysis as a guide."
- "First, did you complete it? If not, then what got in the way? Perhaps you felt embarrassed about your eating and did not want to turn it in. This response to your emotions could interfere with treatment."

- "If you did complete it, the first thing we want to know is what the problem behavior was. This means learning to describe the problem in behavioral terms. Please turn to the path to mindful eating form and, during your 5 minutes, discuss the highest problem behavior that you wrote about during the week."

- "Then, we want you to focus on the key dysfunctional link or links. To clarify, the key dysfunctional link is not the prompting event or the problem behavior. The key dysfunctional link or links is a point at which you capitulated, where you reached the point of no return. Remember, by describing this as a dysfunctional link, we are not judging it. For example, you might identify boredom as a key dysfunctional link in your chain toward a binge. Boredom in and of itself is not dysfunctional. It may be that you need to experience the boredom and not binge. We are calling it a dysfunctional link if your reaction to the link leads you to the problem behavior. The idea is to substitute skills especially at that link so that you don't turn to binge eating [and purging]."

- "Please identify for us the key dysfunctional link or links and what skills you think you'd use next time. If you need help, please ask the group."

Practicing Identifying the Key Dysfunctional Link on the Chain Analysis

Especially in the beginning stages of treatment, it may be difficult for clients to identify the key dysfunctional link or links. In such cases, it may be helpful to use Appendix 3.12 to review typical examples of key dysfunctional links.

The therapists read through the first example:

"In this case, the problem behavior is a 'subjective' binge because the amount of food consumed, as opposed to an 'objective' binge, is not unusually large. The person was walking in a shopping mall and passed a shop selling sweets and confections. That's the prompting event. Looking into the window, the person sensed a physical craving and thought, 'I can't resist them. They're too good.' The emotions identified were anxiety and desire. The person capitulated, experiencing those emotions of anxiety and desire as being too intense to tolerate. This is the key dysfunctional link for that person. Those emotions are not in and of themselves functional or dysfunctional. What is dysfunctional is turning in a driven, out-of-control manner to food to numb yourself or avoid these emotions. In that individual's scenario, we'd spend time in group looking at what happened and what he or she could have done differently. For example, perhaps he or she could have thought about his or her commitment when experiencing the desire and anxiety. This would break the link to the problem behavior."

Therapists might have group members take turns reading through the other examples and discussing the identified links, and so forth. It is important to encourage questions and comments to make sure clients understand the concepts being discussed.

Revisiting the Chain Analysis in Greater Depth

After the brief introduction to the chain analysis and after clients have had the opportunity to fill one out at home, therapists will want to review the chain analysis in greater depth. The therapists underscore how crucial this tool is as a problem-solving strategy for increasing the client's awareness of his or her dysfunctional eating behaviors by allowing detailed examination of the factors that led up to the binge (and purge) and to other problem eating behaviors, as well as of the consequences that followed.

The therapists might begin by reviewing basic information about the chain analysis. Now that the client has attempted one, this information will make more sense. Therapists refer to the figure of the chain at the top of the first page of the chain analysis (Appendix 3.6) to emphasize that problem behaviors such as binge eating (and purging) do not "just happen."

Understandably, as discussed, clients have often engaged in such behaviors so repeatedly that they may feel as if the behavior occurs instantaneously or automatically. With the use of the chain analysis, clients will see more and more clearly how their binge eating (and purging) is actually a learned behavior that can be understood. Prompting events that occur in the environment trigger a set of feelings, thoughts, and actions that lead to the problem eating behavior. The consequences of the problem behavior are important to analyze, too, as they may make it more likely that another binge (and purge) or other problem behavior will occur, thus linking this chain to yet another.

The chain analysis allows clients to slow down the process, to "freeze frame" each link one after the other, so that eventually they can break the chain by substituting more adaptive links than the behaviors they have used in the past.

Ideally, clients would complete the chain as soon as the idea of binge eating and purging occurs or as soon as they notice urges. This would facilitate early identification of factors and might lead to actually breaking the chain. If the problem behavior has already occurred, clients should complete the chain analysis as soon as possible afterward.

In our research studies, we ask clients to fill out a minimum of one chain per week for at least the first 15 sessions. This amount of practice is necessary to give clients sufficient understanding to continue using the tool by themselves once treatment ends. Even if the client does not engage in binge eating (and purging), he or she should use the chain to address another target behavior, either one targeted in the path to mindful eating (Appendix 3.2) or to a problem behavior that is unique to him or her and associated with binge eating. If the client has had absolutely no eating-related problem behaviors in a particular week, he or she might describe a past binge (and/or purge) episode or a non-eating-related problem behavior.

After 15 weeks, clients may fill out chain analyses on an as-needed basis—meaning only if an eating-related problem behavior takes place.

Therapists then review the process of filling out a chain analysis. In a group format, given the complexity of chain analyses, we have found it most time effective to have the group review the sample chain analysis (Appendix 3.6), to elicit one or two client examples from the group to review in detail, or to have the therapists present a typical scenario for the group to work through together. When delivering treatment within 50-minute individual-format sessions, available time is usually sufficient to review the client's actual chain analysis. (Note: The Troubleshooting section on pp. 63–65 offers examples of how to handle clients who do not attempt to fill out a chain analysis.)

For therapists wishing to present a typical scenario to the group, the following has proved useful. Therapists might say: "Let's all work on this scenario. You've had a long day, go to a friend's or family member's dinner party, feel you ate too much at the party, come home, and decide to binge [and purge]. Does that sound like something you've experienced? Let's break it down by going through the chain analysis."

Ask the group to identify the problem behavior (e.g., an objectively large binge [and purge] while at home) and the vulnerability factors (e.g., fatigue after a long day, possibly conflicting feelings about attending the party). Then, lead the group in a discussion regarding identifying the prompting event. The point to emphasize is that there is no right or wrong answer. If a client believes that the event that started him or her on the chain toward the binge (and purge) was the dinner party with its array of tempting foods, then that was the prompting event for that particular client. Other clients might argue that this made them vulnerable but that there was no movement toward binge eating until they were alone, later that night. In that case, the prompting event was being home late at night after the party was over.

Request that clients turn to the second page of the chain analysis (Appendix 3.6) and write down some of the links that would have been included in their own chains, adding, "the smaller and more discrete the links, the better." Typically, clients write down cognitions (e.g., "I shouldn't have eaten so much"), bodily sensations (e.g., feeling uncomfortably full, muscle tension), emotions (e.g., loneliness after the party is over, shame about how much was eaten, regret over something that took place at the party). The therapists then call for ideas from clients about what could have been done differently. Specifically, what more adaptive skills could have been used?

Now have clients look at the third page of the chain. Begin by asking about the immediate and longer term consequences of turning to food to manage the uncomfortable emotions. Clients might identify how the binge (and purge) allowed them to distance themselves from the uncomfortable emotions in the short term but in the longer term led them to feel miserable, defeated, and despondent. Ways to reduce vulnerability may include calming down and taking time to center themselves prior to, during, and after the party—reminding themselves of their commitment to building a truly high quality of life. Ways to prevent the problem event from recurring might include avoiding the kitchen on returning home and going straight to one's bedroom to read, speak on the phone, and/or fill out one's diary card and chain analysis.

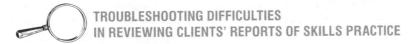

TROUBLESHOOTING DIFFICULTIES IN REVIEWING CLIENTS' REPORTS OF SKILLS PRACTICE

- *Example 1*: The client has completed his or her chain analysis but tends to have great difficulty focusing, during the allotted time of the group session, on identifying the key dysfunctional link.

- *Potential therapist reply*: Note that it is important to distinguish for clients the differences between "telling a story" and reporting from the chain. When story-telling occurs, the therapist should aid the client in focusing on the relevant elements. This can typically be done by saying: "Remember, the key dysfunctional link is the one that you feel is most strongly linked to your problem eating behavior. There is no right or wrong answer. Why don't you turn to page two of your chain analysis and read aloud what you wrote down?"

- *Example 2*: "I didn't fill out my diary card this past week."

- *Potential therapist reply*: "Did you practice any of the skills, even if you didn't circle them on your diary card?" Note that the key here is to distinguish clients who practiced skills but did not record them from clients who did not practice at all. Most clients have at least thought about the skills, and it can be valuable to reinforce this as a means of shaping their behavior. Point out that the diary card is just a way to remind clients to practice skills, and what they did is most important. Then, focus on what got in the way of recording the homework practice (see Example 4).

- *Example 3*: The client did not fill out his or her diary card and/or chain analysis and just binged (and/or purged).

- *Potential therapist reply*: "What do you think is getting in the way of your doing your homework?" Conduct a mini-chain analysis with the client. If the client seems to have difficulty identifying interfering factors, the therapist might ask: "Was it a week from hell? Was it that, at the end of the day, you wanted to forget what you had eaten because you felt embarrassed, not wanting to look at yourself and your behavior? These types of emotions are painful. But what you're bringing up is a very important issue. Your mood and your behavior are tightly linked. Once fear of failure, shame, and embarrassment come in, they can block you from following through on a commitment. How do you get yourself to do something, like practicing skills and filling out your homework sheets, that you don't want to do? We are assuming that you do indeed have some skillful behaviors that you can engage in when you get really anxious, but turning to food is such a knee-jerk response right now that it's the first thing off the shelf. It is crowding out your repertoire of more effective behaviors. Can you recommit right now to really reach for these other skills? And over this next week, can you practice imagining dealing with the feelings and still doing the homework? Capitulating to the urge to avoid means giving yourself up to binge eating [and purging]. Based on your experience, did avoiding doing your homework work help you regulate the uncomfortable emotions you describe?"

- *Example 4*: "I find it overwhelming. I can't figure out exactly what I'm feeling. I can't write it down right."

- *Potential therapist reply*: "Sounds like some capitulating and judging is going on. I think I hear you saying that if you can't get it perfect, you don't want to do it at all? (*Client nods.*) What's great is that you have identified some links that prevent you from being skillful. It is so important not to give up. If something comes up that is making you feel like you want to binge and/or purge but you don't know exactly what it is, that's okay. You can still sit down with the sheets and fill out what you can—even just one link or one of the boxes. It sounds like you got overwhelmed by judging. Sometimes taking a break and focusing on breathing will reduce that so that it's less intense. When you're ready, go back to the diary card or chain and work on one section at a time."

• *Example 5*: "There wasn't a prompting event—nothing was going on. I just started eating."

• *Potential therapist reply*: "Sometimes, when there's no clear prompting event, the issue is the buildup of vulnerability factors. Could that be the case here? What's the thing that if it hadn't happened, you would not have binged? Why did you binge on that day at that time and not at other times?"

• *Example 6*: "I can't figure out whether I had a binge or not."

• *Potential therapist reply*: "This is something I can't tell you—it is something you have to figure out for yourself. It may not be as clear-cut as you'd like, but it depends on an inner experience. Were you out of control while eating? Remember that having conflict about whether to eat or what to eat—that 'should I or shouldn't I' feeling—those do not necessarily mean that you had a binge. Binge eating does not depend on the type of food. Eating nonnutritious food does not necessarily constitute a binge. A binge happens when you feel compelled and out of control, when you can't stop yourself once you start. It's not the same as overeating, feeling as if you were in control but feeling regretful that the amount of food was not consistent with your goals to weigh less. If you determine that you've eaten with a sense of loss of control, the issue is whether you had a very large amount of food or a smaller amount of food. Don't get too hung up on these details."

Dialectical Abstinence

We recommend bringing up the concept of dialectical abstinence, originally developed in DBT for substance abuse (Linehan & Dimeff, 1997),[6] in the second session with the client. It is useful to explain that bringing up this concept had been *planned* as part of the treatment protocol. In other words, therapists are not discussing it because any particular client reported having had a binge (and purge) despite committing to abstinence. It is being brought up now because of its relevance. There simply was not adequate time to review it during the initial session.

Clients coming to treatment are faced with a dilemma. Therapists might say: "You have agreed that you value living up to your potential and feeling fully alive. You recognize that continuing to use food is incompatible with achieving that life and have made a 100% commitment to stopping binge eating [and purging]. The dilemma is that what if, after making that commitment, you had or will have a binge [or purge]?"

To deal effectively with that scenario, clients will be taught a very important and useful concept called dialectical abstinence.

---

[6]Unlike the DBT for substance use disorders model (DBT–SUD), our DBT for BED or BN model does not include the "touchdown every time" concept (e.g., the understanding that clients only are making the commitment for as long as they know with absolute certainty that they can keep it). In our model, the commitment is discussed as a powerful skill in and of itself, even if the client is uncertain about her or his ability to keep it.

"For years, there has been recognition of the existence of opposing forces. The dialectical view is that for every force or position, there exists an opposing force or position, a thesis and an antithesis. A good visual example would be the positive and negative poles on a battery. They can exist side by side but represent polar opposites. A dialectical view searches for a synthesis that is more than the sum of the opposite parts. For example, the yin and yang symbol is black and white, yet the synthesis of these is not merely the color gray. A synthesis transcends both."

The therapists explain that when individuals start to believe in or will see only *one* correct position, *one* way to do things, they tend to get into trouble. The dialectical approach synthesizes the two positions by holding them together. The dialectical approach recognizes that both exist and accepts this synthesis.

"So how does this relate to binge eating [and purging]? It seems very relevant when you understand that we have two opposing forces operating that need to be recognized and reconciled. On the one hand, you have set a goal for yourself to stop binge eating [and purging]. You made a verbal commitment because the reality of the situation is that feeling fully alive and good about yourself is incompatible with binge eating [and purging]. Because the urge to binge [and purge] is so strong, one must have this 100% strong commitment. Anything short would be failure. When faced with the urge to binge [and purge], you cannot have the idea that it is 'OK' to binge [and purge] and fail and to 'just try again.' Such thinking is undermining and will make it more likely that you will decide to binge eat [and purge]."

On the opposite side, it is clear that in not anticipating and preparing for a slip, clients will be less likely to handle such an event effectively, should it occur. "This is the problem we as therapists and you as group members are faced with. How can one deal with these two opposing forces of success and failure? How do you hold onto the goal despite not meeting it? What do we do?" Therapists present the metaphor of the Olympic athlete as a helpful way for clients to think about this, making the following points:

• "Stopping binge eating [and purging] is as big as any major Olympic event. So imagine that you are like Olympic athletes and we, the therapists, are your coaches. For Olympic athletes, absolutely nothing is discussed before the race except winning or 'going for the gold.' If Olympic athletes thought or said that winning a bronze medal 'would be just fine,' then their training mentality, performance, and push would all be affected. That Olympic athlete must also not think about falling down in a race or about what would occur should he or she twist an ankle before the race. Those types of thoughts must stay out of the mind, even though these are possible outcomes, and the athlete must only strive for the gold."
• "In other words, think of yourself as being Olympic athletes in the Stop Binge Eating [and purging] Event. The only thing you can possibly allow yourselves to think about and discuss is absolute and total abstinence."

• "However, using the dialectical view, you, as well as Olympic athletes, must be prepared for the possibility of failure. The dialectical dilemma is that both success and failure exist. The dialectical abstinence solution involves, on the one hand, your 100% certainty that binge eating [and purging] is out of the question and your 100% confidence that you will never binge and/or purge again. However, simultaneously, you must keep in mind—way, way back in the very farthest part so that it never interferes with your resolve—that if you do slip, you will deal with it effectively by accepting it nonjudgmentally and picking yourself back up. This means acknowledging, 'OK, I had a binge [and purge].' You must be able to be aware of the problem and acknowledge it in order to change it. Use the chain analysis, analyze what was going on, become a problem solver. Then recommit to 100% full abstinence, knowing that that was the last time, that you will never slip again."

• "We're saying that it is possible to do these two seemingly contradictory things—commit to absolute abstinence from binge eating [and purging] *and* accept a binge [and purge] should such behavior occur. We are not talking about accepting a binge [and purge] *before* you have one. Saying to yourself, in the back of your mind, 'Oh, I guess it is really OK if I go ahead and binge [and purge] because if I do, I'll just do a chain analysis and recommit,' will undermine your commitment. Instead, this awareness of the possibility of binge eating [and purging] must be buried somewhere outside of your awareness. You'll respond that way if it happens, but as it will never happen, you don't have to worry about it."

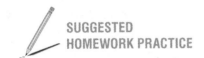

SUGGESTED HOMEWORK PRACTICE

Therapists instruct clients to practice the skill of dialectical abstinence every day, reading over the homework sheet (Appendix 3.13) and filling it out before the next session.

Diaphragmatic Breathing

Inform clients that this next skill, diaphragmatic breathing,[7] will likely be one of the most useful they will learn in this treatment program. Diaphragmatic breathing is deceptively simple. Based on our experience in our research trials, clients report it to be their number-one most frequently used skill. We hear time and again how incredibly helpful clients find it in aiding them to break the chain toward problem eating. For clients who have heard of diaphragmatic breathing or have even practiced it through other modalities (e.g., playing an instrument, yoga), this is an opportunity to strengthen their use of it.

Begin by asking clients to reflect on what happens physically when they experience very strong emotions. Often clients report that their breathing changes, becoming dysregulated, and their heart rates speed up. Clients may also notice dizziness. Point out that such physical sensations can increase feelings of distress and

---

[7]The method taught for diaphragmatic breathing is similar to that taught by Barlow and Craske (2006) in *Mastery of Your Anxiety and Panic.*

cause clients to want to stop these feelings by turning to binge eating (and purging). Deep breathing interrupts this physical process and can reduce emotional distress. Furthermore, deep breathing can facilitate mindfulness, a state of mind that will be discussed in the Mindfulness module. One purpose of mindfulness is to strengthen clients' ability to focus attention and increase their awareness of the present moment. Maintaining attention on a particular focus, such as the breath, is one means of practicing mindfulness. The purpose of this focus is to bring the attention back to the "here and now," using a focus on breath as the anchor.

Therapists might state:

> "Learning and practicing deep breathing and focusing on your breath are very helpful for relieving emotional distress and physical tensions that have built up and may trigger your urges to binge [and purge]. Your breath is always with you, so the skill of deep breathing is a readily available skill, always right under your nose. When you feel an urge to binge [and purge], you can calm yourself down and ride out the urge by breathing. In doing so, you are replacing the problematic eating behavior and thoughts with deep breathing and a focus on your breath."

Therapists might find it helpful to use the following script, modifying as needed.

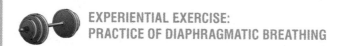

EXPERIENTIAL EXERCISE: PRACTICE OF DIAPHRAGMATIC BREATHING

"Put one hand on your abdomen and one on your chest. This isn't about trying to do anything fancy! Just notice your hand on your abdomen. Then breathe while having your hand on your abdomen. Practice taking slow, regular, flowing breaths so that the hand on your abdomen moves up and down and the hand on your chest is still. [Note: Therapists may find it useful to demonstrate, for example: "If you want to watch me, it is like this."] Remember, you are just doing slow breathing. Focus on the hand on your abdomen slowing moving up and down. Be patient. If you notice you are not breathing from your diaphragm, try not to judge yourself. Just keep your awareness on your breath, letting it flow in and out. Your mind *will* wander, but the more you practice the easier it will be to notice that and just bring your mind back to your breath.

"Inhale and exhale through your nose. As you inhale, slowly count *one, two, three*. As you exhale, silently say to yourself something such as, 'Relax' or 'Calm down.' Do this while counting up to 10 and then start at 1 again. Try to keep your awareness on your breath. If it's helpful to think of it this way, the rate of breathing is usually about 10–12 breaths per minute. That means taking about 3 seconds to slowly inhale and 3 seconds to slowly exhale.

"You can use this skill when you have worries or anxiety or any time you notice your emotions becoming more intense. Simply slow down and focus on your breath. In addition to practicing this skill when you are feeling intense emotions, practice it regularly when nothing is going on—so that you gain facility with the skill. The more you practice using this skill, the more you'll be aware of your mind and your breath. The breath can serve as the anchor to the mind."

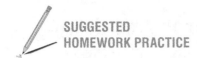

SUGGESTED
HOMEWORK PRACTICE

1. Therapists instruct clients to practice diaphragmatic breathing twice a day for about 3–5 minutes at a time—when the sole purpose is to practice. This is called formal practice.

2. In addition, therapists instruct clients to practice informally—such as when they are driving, while at a party, while on the phone, while at work.

3. Therapists should make clear that it is especially important for clients to practice using this skill when noticing any urges to binge eat (and purge).

4. Clients should mark their practice of this skill on their diary cards by circling "diaphragmatic breathing" each day they use it.

Emotion Dysregulation Model of Problem Eating

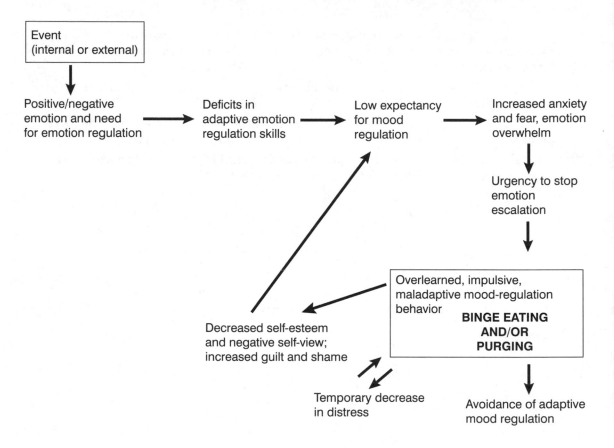

Goals of Treatment, Goals of Skills Training, and Treatment Targets

Treatment Goals: Stop problematic eating behaviors (e.g., binge eating, binge–purge episodes).

Goals of Skills Training: Learn and practice adaptive emotion regulation skills to replace maladaptive binge eating and other problem eating behaviors.

Treatment Targets:

PATH TO MINDFUL EATING

1. Stop any behavior that interferes with treatment.*

2. Stop binge eating (and purging).

3. Eliminate mindless eating.

4. Decrease cravings, urges, preoccupation with food.

5. Decrease capitulating—that is, closing off options to not binge eat (and purge).

6. Decrease apparently irrelevant behaviors—for example, buying binge foods "for company."

INCREASE SKILLFUL EMOTION REGULATION BEHAVIORS[†] BY LEARNING AND PRACTICING:

MINDFULNESS SKILLS

EMOTION REGULATION SKILLS

DISTRESS TOLERANCE SKILLS

Following the path to mindful eating will naturally lead to healthy weight regulation and an enhanced quality of life.

*This path to mindful eating hierarchy is based on the population of clients recruited for our research trials. Though not explicitly delineated in this model, decreasing any life-threatening behaviors takes precedence over the other targets, just as in standard DBT, if crises arise.
[†]Skillful emotion regulation behaviors include skills taught in all the standard DBT modules. The term "emotion regulation skills" in this context is not meant to apply to only the Emotion Regulation Skills module.

Group Member Treatment Agreements

1. I agree that I will keep confidential the information discussed during group sessions, including the names of other group members.

2. I agree not to form private relationships with other group members outside of the group sessions.

3. I agree to arrive at sessions on time.

4. I agree to attend sessions each week and to stay for the entire 2-hour session.

5. I agree to call ahead of time if I will miss or be late for a session. If I miss a session, I agree to come to the clinic to listen to the recorded (e.g., audiotaped or videotaped) session and to complete the skills practice and share this practice during the homework review.

6. I agree to practice the skills taught.

7. I agree to do my absolute best to stop binge eating and to help other group members to stop binge eating.

8. I agree to complete the homework assignments and bring them with me to each session.

9. [Note: If applicable] I agree to complete the research questionnaires and interviews that are part of this treatment program.

Group member's signature _____ Date _____

Individual Client Treatment Agreements

1. I agree to arrive at sessions on time.

2. I agree to attend sessions each week and to stay for the entire 50-minute session.

3. I agree to call ahead of time if I will miss or be late for a session.

4. I agree to practice the skills taught.

5. I agree to do my absolute best to stop binge eating and purging.

6. I agree to complete the homework assignments and bring them with me to each session.

7. [Note: If applicable] I agree to complete the research questionnaires and interviews that are part of this treatment program.

Client's signature _____ Date _____

Therapist Treatment Agreements

1. I agree that I will keep confidential the information discussed, including the [names of group members] or [client's name].

2. [Note: If applicable] I agree not to form private relationships with other group members outside of group sessions.

3. I agree to arrive at sessions on time.

4. I agree to attend sessions each week and to stay for the entire [2-hour] or [50-minute] session.

5. I agree to inform the group if I will miss or be late for a session. [If applicable] If I miss a session I agree to listen to the recorded (e.g., audiotaped or videotaped) session.

6. I agree to practice the skills taught.

7. I agree to do my absolute best to deliver the best treatment that I can to help [group members] or [the client] stop binge eating [and purging].

_____   _____
Cotherapist's signature   Date

_____   _____
[Cotherapist's signature]   [Date]

Sample Chain Analysis

Behavioral Chain Analysis of Problem Behavior: Page 1

Name: _____ Date filled out: _____ Date of problem behavior: _____

VULNERABILITY

PROBLEM BEHAVIOR

PROMPTING EVENT

LINKS

CONSEQUENCES

WHAT EXACTLY IS THE MAJOR *PROBLEM BEHAVIOR* THAT I AM ANALYZING?

One-hour binge on a variety of junk foods from convenience store.

WHAT PROMPTING EVENT *IN THE ENVIRONMENT* STARTED ME ON THE CHAIN TO MY PROBLEM BEHAVIOR? Start Day: __Monday__

My husband and I got into an argument because he went against our agreement that his mother would stay in a hotel during the holidays. Instead, he told his mother that she could stay at our house after all.

WHAT THINGS IN MYSELF AND MY ENVIRONMENT MADE ME *VULNERABLE?*
Start Day: __Saturday__

I felt stressed and overwhelmed at all I had included on my to-do list (grocery shopping, polishing silverware, getting house in order, washing dog, washing car). I was irritated at my husband for not helping. I had not gotten enough sleep and felt exhausted and irritable. Over the years, I have developed the pattern of using binge eating when upset.

Behavioral Chain Analysis of Problem Behavior: Page 2

Name: _____   Date filled out: _____

LINKS OF BEHAVIOR (actions; body sensations; cognitions; feelings) and EVENTS

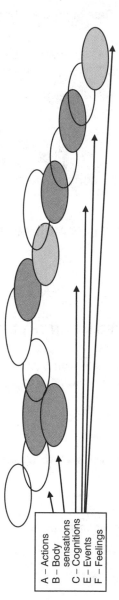

A – Actions
B – Body sensations
C – Cognitions
E – Events
F – Feelings

LINK—ACTUAL	ABC–EF	NEW SKILLFUL ABC–EF
1. Grabbed my things and stormed out of the house.	A	Noticed urge to "do" something and ride the wave of the urge without acting on it.
2. Thought about the argument. Wondered if I should go home and apologize.	C	Observe. Just notice. Don't judge thoughts or hang onto them or push them away.
3. Felt sad as I thought about the holidays and how complicated it had all become.	F	Be mindful of my current emotion. Don't try to block it. Accept. Be open to my sadness. What is its function?
4. Felt muscles tighten up and gripped the steering wheel. Started driving faster.	B	Find a safe place to pull off the road and do diaphragmatic breathing.
5. Thought "I don't care anymore. I'll show him. I won't come home for hours."	C	Find my Wise Mind. What do I value in my heart of hearts? Wise Mind guides me to work this out.
6. Began thinking about getting food and what I would choose, how much better I would feel if I ate.	C	Observe the pull to give up. Observe the way I pretend I'll feel better. Observe the need to self-soothe. Self-soothe by listening to the radio.
7. Pulled into convenience store and bought binge foods.	A	Remind myself of my commitment to stop using binge eating as a solution. Recommit, in this moment, distract with activities: going to store and buying a magazine, crossword puzzle, or lottery ticket.

Adapted from Marsha M. Linehan. Copyright 1996–2009. Adapted with permission in *Dialectical Behavior Therapy for Binge Eating and Bulimia* by Debra L. Safer, Christy F. Telch, and Eunice Y. Chen (2009). Permission to photocopy this appendix is granted to purchasers of this book for personal use only (see copyright page for details).

Name: _____ Date filled out: _____

WHAT EXACTLY WERE THE *CONSEQUENCES* IN THE ENVIRONMENT?

1. When I returned home it was harder to talk with my husband.

2.

AND IN MYSELF?

1. Immediately after all the food was gone, I felt exhausted yet relieved. The thoughts and feelings about the fight felt a distant memory, not important. Just wanted to go home and sleep.

2. Once I got home I felt guilty because I didn't want to do anything but go to bed. My stomach was upset. Felt sick and self-hating. Ashamed.

WAYS TO REDUCE MY *VULNERABILITY* IN THE FUTURE

First, I can decrease my level of stress and tension by reducing the demands I place on myself. I can also focus on the pleasure and satisfaction I derive from some of the "tasks" I set for myself. Second, I can ask others for help and communicate my feelings rather than expect them to read my mind.

WAYS TO PREVENT *PRECIPITATING EVENT* FROM HAPPENING AGAIN

Discuss with my husband "rules" for talking about areas of conflict and disagreement. For example, only talking when we both agree on the timing, genuinely listening to each other's position, agreeing to end the discussion and return to it later if it is at an impasse or is escalating.

WHAT *HARM* DID MY PROBLEM BEHAVIOR CAUSE?

The greatest harm was to myself. I felt ashamed and worthless after the binge. Physically sick. I noticed I withdrew from my husband and was less able to solve the real issues at hand.

PLANS TO *REPAIR, CORRECT,* AND *OVERCORRECT* THE HARM

I will apologize to myself and commit to never, ever binge eating again. I will make a promise from deep within to stop, observe, describe, and use all of the skills I can next time the binge chain starts. Apologize to my husband for my role in the fighting and suggest we do something we both enjoy. I will overcorrect by donating canned food at the grocery store for the needy.

MY DEEPEST THOUGHTS AND FEELINGS ABOUT THIS (THAT I WANT TO SHARE)

In my heart of hearts, my wise self, I know that this is not how I want to behave or conduct my life. I am reacting rather than taking the time to understand, explore, or examine the thoughts and feelings evoked. I miss out on knowing my experience, knowing who I am. I blur my experience with binge eating. This deeply saddens me. I want to stop binge eating.

Guidelines for Filling Out a Behavioral Chain Analysis of a Problem Behavior

1. **Problem behavior**: Specify the problem behavior (e.g., not practicing skills, binge eating [large or small], binge eating and purging, mindless eating) in the space provided on the first page of the chain. Be specific and detailed in describing characteristics of the behavior.

2. **Prompting event**: In the box on the first page, fill in the specific event that started the whole chain or sequence of events leading to the problem behavior. Always start with an action or an event in your environment even if it doesn't seem to you that the environmental event "caused" the problem behavior. Examples of prompting events might be weighing yourself, looking in the mirror, attending a buffet dinner, being asked to volunteer on a committee, and so forth. The prompting can be anything or everything that was happening at the moment you started off on the path to your problem behavior. Describe, as well, what was going on inside of you when the prompting event started (e.g., what you were doing, thinking, feeling).

3. **Vulnerability factors**: Identify in general what factors (both in yourself and in the environment) occurred before the prompting event that made you more vulnerable to it. In other words, what gave the prompting event such power? These factors might include those within you—such as physical illness, unbalanced eating or sleeping, use of drugs or alcohol, emotions (e.g., sadness, anger, fear, loneliness), or behaviors (e.g., inactivity or procrastination). Or they might be factors in your environment—either positive or negative—such as availability of tempting foods, being alone, increased demands at home or at work, and so forth.

4. **Links in the chain**: On the second page of the chain, write out the main links in the chain that hooked the prompting event to the problem behavior. Notice what comes first: the sensation? Feeling? Thought? Describe the links in the sequence they occur. Links might include actions or things that you did (e.g., yelled at your child or partner, stopped at grocery store), body sensations (e.g., knot in stomach), cognitions or thoughts (e.g., "I'm too fat," "None of my clothes look good," "I'll never get this done," "I can't wait"), events (e.g., boss asked me to stay late, invited to a pot-luck dinner), and feelings (e.g., angry, overwhelmed, lonely, scared).

5. **New skillful solutions**: On the lines in the second column, describe the specific skills that you could have used to replace the link and break the chain of events leading to the problem behavior. Sometimes it is helpful to fill these in with a different colored pen or pencil.

6. **Consequences**: On p. 3 in the top box, describe the consequences of the problem behavior, both in the environment and in yourself. The idea is to identify the consequences that *reinforce* the problem behavior, making it more likely to happen again. Describe both the immediate consequences (e.g., an increased sense of power over others, deciding not to attend a party, feeling numb, no longer anxious about an argument), as well as the longer-term consequences (e.g., depressed mood, physical discomfort, weight gain).

7. **Ways to reduce your vulnerability in the future**: Describe in detail ways you can prevent the chain of events from starting by reducing your vulnerability to the chain of events (e.g., improved sleep, not purchasing large quantities of food, balancing work with relaxation).

8. **Ways to prevent precipitating event from happening again**: Describe the things you can do to prevent the prompting event from happening again. For example, one might make an agreement with a partner to take a time out before an argument escalates. Then, follow through on this agreement.

9. **What harm did your problem behavior cause?** Describe in detail the damage or harm your problem behavior caused for you and others. How did it affect your self-confidence? Your belief in your ability to maintain control over yourself for your long-term best interests? Your relationships with others?

10. **Plan to repair**: Describe what you will do to repair the harm that resulted from the problem behavior (e.g., what will you do to correct the blow to your self-confidence or the damage to relationships that the problem behavior caused?).

11. **Deepest thoughts and feelings about this (that you want to share)**: Spend some time encouraging and allowing your deepest thoughts and feelings to surface about this chain of events and problem behavior. Write down the thoughts and feelings that you want to share.

Chain Analysis

Behavioral Chain Analysis of Problem Behavior: Page 1

Name: _____   Date filled out: _____   Date of problem behavior: _____

WHAT EXACTLY IS THE MAJOR *PROBLEM BEHAVIOR* THAT I AM ANALYZING?

WHAT PROMPTING EVENT *IN THE ENVIRONMENT* STARTED ME ON THE CHAIN TO MY PROBLEM BEHAVIOR? Start Day: _____

WHAT THINGS IN MYSELF AND MY ENVIRONMENT MADE ME *VULNERABLE*? Start Day: _____

Behavioral Chain Analysis of Problem Behavior: Page 2

Name: _____   Date filled out: _____

LINKS OF BEHAVIOR (actions; body sensations; cognitions; feelings) and EVENTS

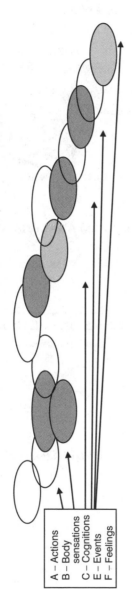

A – Actions
B – Body sensations
C – Cognitions
E – Events
F – Feelings

LINK—ACTUAL	ABC–EF	NEW SKILLFUL ABC–EF
1.	A	
2.	C	
3.	F	
4.	B	
5.	C	
6.	C	
7.	A	

80

Behavioral Chain Analysis of Problem Behavior: Page 3

Name: _____ Date filled out: _____

WHAT EXACTLY WERE THE *CONSEQUENCES* IN THE ENVIRONMENT?

1.

2.

AND IN MYSELF?

1.

2.

WAYS TO REDUCE MY *VULNERABILITY* IN THE FUTURE

WAYS TO PREVENT *PRECIPITATING EVENT* FROM HAPPENING AGAIN

WHAT *HARM* DID MY PROBLEM BEHAVIOR CAUSE?

PLANS TO *REPAIR, CORRECT,* AND *OVERCORRECT* THE HARM

MY DEEPEST THOUGHTS AND FEELINGS ABOUT THIS (THAT I WANT TO SHARE)

APPENDIX 3.9

Diary Card

Front Side of Diary Card

DIARY CARD For week beginning: Mon Tue Wed Thur Fri Sat Sun (circle one) On date: ___ / ___ / ___									Please write in your user ID or initials _____						This week I filled out this side of the diary card ___ each day ___ 4–6 times ___ 2–3 times ___ once	Urge to quit therapy (0–6): Before therapy session ___ After therapy session ___	
Day	Urge to Binge (0–6)*	Urge to Purge (0–6)*	How many times (if any) did you ...? Binge	Purge	Mindless Eating How many times?	Any AIBs?† Apparently irrelevant behaviors? Did you set yourself up? (Circle one)	Did you capitulate? Give in or surrender? (0–6)*	Food cravings?* (0–6)*	Preoccupied with food? (0–6)*	ANGER (0–6)*	SADNESS (0–6)*	Fear/Anxiety (0–6)*	SHAME (0–6)*	PRIDE (0–6)*	HAPPINESS (0–6)*	Rate how much you used the skills (0–7)‡
Mon						Yes No										
Tue						Yes No										
Wed						Yes No										
Thur						Yes No										
Fri						Yes No										
Sat						Yes No										
Sun						Yes No										

Date Weighed ___ / ___ / ___ Weight _____

*Please rate from 0 to 6 the highest rating for the day (0 = did not experience the urge/thought/feeling, to 6 = experienced the urge/thought/feeling intensely)

†Describe AIBs.

‡USED SKILL

0 = Not thought about or used

1 = Thought about, not used, didn't want to

2 = Thought about, not used, wanted to

3 = Tried but couldn't use them

4 = Tried, could use them, but they didn't help

5 = Tried, could use them, helped

6 = Used skills without trying, didn't help

7 = Used skills without trying, helped

Skills Practice Record (Reverse Side of Diary Card)

SKILLS DIARY CARD	Instructions: Circle the days you worked on each skill.	How often did you fill out this side? ___ Daily ___ 4–6x ___ 2–3x ___ Once					
1. Commitment	Mon	Tues	Wed	Thurs	Fri	Sat	Sun
2. 3" × 5" card	Mon	Tues	Wed	Thurs	Fri	Sat	Sun
3. Diaphragmatic Breathing	Mon	Tues	Wed	Thurs	Fri	Sat	Sun
4. Wise Mind	Mon	Tues	Wed	Thurs	Fri	Sat	Sun
5. Observe: Just noticing	Mon	Tues	Wed	Thurs	Fri	Sat	Sun
6. Describe: Just putting words to	Mon	Tues	Wed	Thurs	Fri	Sat	Sun
7. Participate: Entering into the experience	Mon	Tues	Wed	Thurs	Fri	Sat	Sun
8. Mindful Eating	Mon	Tues	Wed	Thurs	Fri	Sat	Sun
9. Nonjudgmental Stance	Mon	Tues	Wed	Thurs	Fri	Sat	Sun
10. One-Mindfully: In the moment	Mon	Tues	Wed	Thurs	Fri	Sat	Sun
11. Effectively: Focus on what works	Mon	Tues	Wed	Thurs	Fri	Sat	Sun
12. Urge Surfing	Mon	Tues	Wed	Thurs	Fri	Sat	Sun
13. Alternate Rebellion	Mon	Tues	Wed	Thurs	Fri	Sat	Sun
14. Mindfulness of Your Current Emotion (Observe/Describe)	Mon	Tues	Wed	Thurs	Fri	Sat	Sun
15. Loving Your Emotions	Mon	Tues	Wed	Thurs	Fri	Sat	Sun
16. Identify Your Emotion(s)	Mon	Tues	Wed	Thurs	Fri	Sat	Sun
17. Function of Emotion(s)	Mon	Tues	Wed	Thurs	Fri	Sat	Sun
18. Reduce Vulnerability	Mon	Tues	Wed	Thurs	Fri	Sat	Sun
19. Build Mastery	Mon	Tues	Wed	Thurs	Fri	Sat	Sun
20. Build Positive Experiences	Mon	Tues	Wed	Thurs	Fri	Sat	Sun
21. Mindful of Positive Experiences	Mon	Tues	Wed	Thurs	Fri	Sat	Sun
22. Opposite-to-Emotion Action	Mon	Tues	Wed	Thurs	Fri	Sat	Sun
23. Observing Your Breath	Mon	Tues	Wed	Thurs	Fri	Sat	Sun
24. Half-Smiling	Mon	Tues	Wed	Thurs	Fri	Sat	Sun
25. Awareness Exercises	Mon	Tues	Wed	Thurs	Fri	Sat	Sun
26. Radical Acceptance (Turning the Mind, Willingness)	Mon	Tues	Wed	Thurs	Fri	Sat	Sun
27. Burning Your Bridges	Mon	Tues	Wed	Thurs	Fri	Sat	Sun
28. Distract	Mon	Tues	Wed	Thurs	Fri	Sat	Sun
29. Self-Soothe	Mon	Tues	Wed	Thurs	Fri	Sat	Sun
30. Improve the Moment	Mon	Tues	Wed	Thurs	Fri	Sat	Sun
31. Pros and Cons	Mon	Tues	Wed	Thurs	Fri	Sat	Sun
32. Coping Ahead	Mon	Tues	Wed	Thurs	Fri	Sat	Sun
33. Did Not Practice/Use Any Skills	Mon	Tues	Wed	Thurs	Fri	Sat	Sun

Instructions for Filling Out a Diary Card

Completing your diary card on a daily basis is an essential component of your treatment. "Mindful" completion of the diary card (i.e., paying attention *without* judging) increases awareness of what is going on for you. Therefore, completing the diary card is a skillful behavior. You will derive the greatest benefit if you complete the diary card on a daily basis. We suggest you complete it at the end of each day, but if another time is more convenient for you, that is fine. Here's how you complete the card:

Initials/ID: Write in your initials (or ID# if participating in a research protocol).

How often did you fill out this side? Place a check mark to indicate how frequently you filled in the diary card during the past week.

Day and date: Write in the calendar date (month/day/year) under each day of the week.

Urge to binge: Refer to the legend and choose the number from the scale (0–6) that best represents your highest rating for the day. The key characteristics of the urge to consider when making your rating are intensity (how strongly you felt the urge) and duration (how long the urge lasted).

Urge to purge: Refer to the legend and choose the number from the scale (0–6) that best represents your highest rating for the day. The key characteristics of the urge to consider when making your rating are intensity (how strongly you felt the urge) and duration (how long the urge lasted).

Binge episodes: Write the number of binge episodes you had each day, if any. A binge refers to an eating episode in which you felt a loss of control while eating, as if you could not stop. Large (or "objective") binge episodes refer to amounts of food that are unquestionably larger than most people would eat under similar circumstances. Some guidelines include eating two full meals or more or three or more entrees/main courses. Other examples would include one-half box of cookies and a quart of ice cream. Small (or "subjective") binge episodes involve feeling out of control when eating an amount of food that most people would not consider large or excessive, even if you would (e.g., candy bar, one-half bag of microwave popcorn).

Purge episodes: Write the number of episodes in which you used vomiting or other behaviors (e.g., laxatives, fasting) as a means to compensate for food eaten.

Mindless eating: Write in the number of "mindless" eating episodes that you had each day. Mindless eating refers to not paying attention to what you are eating, although you do not feel the sense of loss of control that you do during binge episodes. A typical example of mindless eating would be sitting in front of the TV and eating a bag of microwave popcorn or chips without any awareness of the eating (i.e., somehow, the food was gone, and you were only vaguely aware of having eaten it). Again, however, you didn't feel a sense of being out of control during the eating.

(continued)

Apparently irrelevant behaviors (AIBs): Circle either "yes" or "no" depending on whether you did or did not have any AIBs that day. If you did, briefly describe the AIB in the place provided or on another sheet of paper. An AIB refers to behaviors that, on first glance, do not seem relevant to binge eating and purging but that actually are important in the behavior chain leading to these behaviors. You may convince yourself that the behavior doesn't matter or really won't affect your goal to stop bingeing and purging when, in fact, the behavior matters a great deal. A typical AIB might be buying several boxes of your favorite Girl Scout cookies because you wanted to help out a neighbor's daughter (of course, you could buy the cookies and donate them to the neighbor).

Capitulating: Refer to the legend and choose the number from the scale (0–6) that best represents your highest rating for the day. The key characteristics to consider when making your rating are intensity (strength of the capitulating) and duration (how long it lasted). Capitulating refers to giving up on your goals to stop binge eating and to skillfully cope with emotions. Instead, you capitulate or surrender to bingeing, acting as if there is no other option or way to cope than with food.

Preoccupied with food: Refer to the legend and choose the number from the scale (0–6) that best represents your highest rating for the day. Food preoccupation refers to your thoughts or attention being absorbed or focused on food. For example, your thoughts of a dinner party and the presence of your favorite foods may absorb your attention so much that you have trouble concentrating at work.

Emotion columns: Refer to the legend and choose the number from the scale (0–6) that best represents your highest rating for the day. The key characteristics to consider when making your rating are intensity (strength of the emotion) and duration (how long it lasted).

Used skills: Refer to the legend and choose the number from the scale (0–7) that best represents your attempts to use the skills each day. When making your rating, consider whether or not you thought about using any of the skills that day, whether or not you actually used any of the skills, and whether or not the skills helped.

Weight: Weigh yourself once each week and record your weight in pounds in the space provided. Please write in the date you weighed yourself. It is best if you choose the same day each week to weigh yourself. Many clients find that arriving a few minutes early to the session and weighing themselves at the clinic is a good way to remember to do this.

Urge to quit therapy: Indicate the strength of your urge to quit therapy before the session and after the session each week. Both of these ratings should be made for the same session as the one in which you received the diary card. It is best to make both of these ratings as soon as possible following that day's session. Use a 0–6 scale of intensity of the urge, with 0 indicating no urge to quit and a 6 indicating the strongest urge to quit.

Completing the skills side of the diary card:

How often did you fill out this side? Place a check mark to indicate how frequently you filled out the skills side of the diary card during the week.

Skills practice: Go down the column for each day of the week and circle each skill that you practiced or used that day. If you did not practice or use any of the skills that particular day, then circle that day on the last line, which states, "Did not practice/use any skills."

Structuring Client's Report of Skills Practice

1. Did you have a binge?
2. Did you practice the skills?
    a. If no, what got in the way?
    b. If yes, what worked?
3. Did you fill out your diary card and chain analysis?
    a. If not, what got in the way?
    b. If yes,
        i. What was the problem behavior?
        ii. What was the dysfunctional link?
Skills Taught Thus Far
1. Practicing the commitment
2. 3″ × 5″ card
3. Filling out diary card and chain analysis

Sample Chains Focusing on Key Dysfunctional Link(s)

Example 1	ABC–EF	Substitute Skills Here
Saw shop selling sweets at mall	Event (*prompting event*)	
Sensed physical craving	**B**odily Sensation	
"I can't resist them"; "They're too good."	**C**ognition	
Desire, Anxiety	Emotion (key dysfunctional link)	
Subjective binge (and purge) on sweets	Action (*problem behavior*)	

Example 2	ABC–EF	Substitute Skills Here
Argument with partner or friend	Event	
Anger	Emotion	
"I'll show them!"	**C**ognition (key dysfunctional link)	
Objective binge (and purge)	Action (*problem behavior*)	

Example 3	ABC–EF	Substitute Skills Here
Didn't get something you wanted. Someone let you down.	Event (*prompting event*)	
"I didn't know this could hurt so much."	Cognition	
"I can't handle this. It's too much. I'm out of control."	Cognition	
Demoralization/Despair	Emotion (key dysfunctional link)	
Objective binge (and purge)	Action	

Example 4	ABC–EF	Substitute Skills Here
At a buffet	Event (*prompting event*)	
Ate more than planned	Action	
"I can't believe I didn't have more control."	Cognition	
Shame	Emotion (key dysfunctional link)	
Subjective binge (and purge)	Action (*problem behavior*)	

Dialectical Abstinence

Dialectical Abstinence

The dialectical view recognizes that for every force or position there exists an opposing force or position: a thesis and antithesis; the yin and the yang. A dialectical view searches for a synthesis that is more than the sum of the opposite parts. For example, the yin and yang symbol is black and white, yet the synthesis of these is not merely the color gray. A synthesis transcends both.

On the one hand, you've made a 100% commitment to stop bingeing, and anything short would be a failure. When faced with the urge to binge, you cannot have the idea that it is "OK" to binge and fail and to "just try again." Such thinking would undermine your goals and make it more likely that you will decide to binge eat. On the other hand, you need to be prepared to deal with a binge effectively if it does occur. You can create the synthesis by recognizing that both forces exist. In the forefront of your mind is your awareness of your 100% commitment and 100% certainty that binge eating is not an option. However, simultaneously, way, way back in the very farthest part, so that it never interferes with your resolve, is the awareness that if you slip, you will deal with it effectively by figuring out what happened, accepting it, not judging yourself, and picking yourself back up and concentrating on what you have learned. Then you recommit to stopping bingeing, back to the 100% knowledge that you will never slip again. The dialectical abstinence solution involves holding the two opposite forces: 100% certainty that binge eating is out of the question and the resolve to deal with it effectively if it happens.

A good mental picture is an Olympic athlete. When the athlete is training, nothing is discussed except winning and going for the gold. If the Olympian athlete thought or said that winning a bronze medal would be fine, then his or her training mentality and performance would be affected. The athlete is similar to you in that you can focus only on absolute and total binge abstinence. Yet, of course, you must also be prepared for the possibility of failure, and the key is to be prepared to fail well.

It is also useful to apply a dialectical view toward yourself. You have come into therapy to make a change so that you can live the high-quality life that you want. At the same time, you must accept yourself just as you are, in this moment. Otherwise, you put yourself into a state of self-criticism, self-loathing, and self-aversion—a state in which it's very easy to feel hopeless, to give up, and to experience urges to binge eat. A dialectical view involves accepting exactly where you are, right at this moment. It doesn't mean necessarily approving of where you are or liking it. But it means accepting it the way you accept gravity. It simply is your reality at this moment. The synthesis is that in accepting yourself exactly as you are *in this moment*, you are doing something you most likely have never been able to do. Accepting yourself as you are, without judgment, means you have already begun to change.

Instructions for Practicing Dialectical Abstinence

Practice allowing yourself to know that success and failure can exist simultaneously. Make a **100% commitment to stop binge eating** and also reserve in the back of your mind that if you slip you'll deal with it effectively. Keep one in the forefront of your mind and the other far back, so far back that it doesn't interfere with your resolve. If you do slip, practice accepting the slip, not judging yourself, picking yourself up again, and recommitting to your 100% resolve to never binge again. Remember, commitment is an active process. It involves continual awareness and recommitment. Write about your practice of this skill in the following space (or reverse side).

CHAPTER 4

Mindfulness Core Skills

Mindfulness skills are taught at the beginning of treatment because they are the basic or core skills that clients need to learn in order to successfully utilize the other skills taught over the course of treatment. Mindfulness skills form the foundation on which the other skills are built. That is, when clients are firmly rooted in Mindfulness, they can see more clearly what constitutes skillful behavior and, therefore, which skills to use. In its broadest sense, mindfulness is simply keeping something in mind (e.g., the breath) or being aware or noticing what is happening (e.g., being tired). This ability to keep something in mind, to notice or be aware, is fundamental to deciding what skillful action to take. Therefore, Mindfulness skills are the foundation on which clients must stand to skillfully regulate emotions. All human beings possess the ability to be mindful; all have the seed of mindfulness within them. Most need to water the seed through daily Mindfulness practice, so the seed can be strengthened and grow from a seed into a tree that provides shelter.

The first step in orienting clients to the Mindfulness skills (Appendix 4.1) is to state unequivocally that these skills are essential, fundamental, and key to their achieving their desired goals of stopping binge eating (and purging) and experiencing a happier, less stressful quality of life. That is, therapists must convincingly sell clients on the fundamental nature of Mindfulness skills and link them to stopping binge eating (and purging), as well as to improving the client's quality of life. The importance of emphasizing Mindfulness skills cannot be overstated. Clients may assume that mindfulness is some abstract concept that they cannot possibly learn or practice. Therapists must reassure clients that mindfulness, or paying attention in a particular way, is a skill everyone can develop. A brief review of the DBT emotion regulation model of problem eating (Chapter 3, Appendix 3.1) may facilitate making links between learning the Mindfulness skills, emotion regulation, and stopping binge eating (and purging). This model conceptualizes binge eating, purging, mindless eating, preoccupations with food, and all other problem eating behaviors as attempts to cope with emotions that feel out of control and overwhelming. The link between emotions and behavior becomes so overlearned that clients are frequently unaware of the emotions that trigger their maladaptive eating patterns. Turning to food in response to emotion dysregulation often feels automatic, like a knee-jerk reaction. This is where the mindfulness skills fit in. These are awareness skills that empower clients to break the automatic link between emotions and problem eating, for example, by noticing that feeling discouraged leads to the urge to binge.

Mindfulness skills enable clients to experience emotions as arising and passing away rather than reacting emotionally by binge eating (and purging). Mindfulness skills teach clients to experience emotions without judging them or reacting to them in a manner that ends up backfiring and creating more pain and suffering. Though clients will be taught other modules, they will continue to practice Mindfulness throughout the treatment and, hopefully, for the rest of their lives. These skills form the bedrock supporting clients in learning to master mental processes (e.g., attention) that facilitate adaptive emotion regulation rather than experiencing their minds as beyond their own control. When introducing Mindfulness skills, therapists will want to emphasize both that these skills take time, patience, and practice to learn and will not offer an "instant fix" *and* that clients *can* learn these skills and receive some benefit even at the beginning of practice. It will not be magic and instantly solve all problems, but practicing Mindfulness will help by building an adaptive skill and weakening the habit of binge eating. As with anything worth having, to get something out of these skills requires an investment. Successfully developing Mindfulness will require the clients' commitment, perseverance, intention, effort, and continued practice over their lifetimes.

Therapists might liken practicing Mindfulness skills to going to the gym. Regular practice is required to build muscle. The benefits of strong muscles, like those of Mindfulness, transfer from the gym to many aspects of a client's life. And if clients stop going to the gym, muscles deteriorate. Like learning to ride a bicycle or to dance salsa, practicing Mindfulness may feel awkward initially. But in the end, clients should be able to access Mindfulness skills without effort—in the way that, with lots of practice, one "becomes" the bicycle or "becomes" the dance.

DEFINITIONS OF MINDFULNESS

A good place to begin the discussion of Mindfulness is to provide clients with several definitions (see Marlatt, 1994, pp. 176–177). These definitions can be read aloud to the group while clients follow along on a printed copy that clients may also review at home. To be mindful is to keep something in mind, to pay attention. For example, if you are told "Be mindful of how you speak," you are being asked to pay attention, to be aware of what you are saying and how you are saying it. Similarly, being mindful of one's emotions involves keeping emotions in mind, being aware, paying attention. Mindfulness is often defined as being nonjudgmental and "present moment." In other words, the awareness or attention is nonjudgmental and present oriented. It is important to underscore, as noted, that developing this type of attention or awareness takes effort and practice.

Mindfulness is that quality of attention which notices without choosing, without preference. It is a choice-less awareness that, like the sun, shines on all things equally. (Goldstein & Kornfield, 1987, p. 19)

So Mindfulness is simply noticing what is happening, what is arising and passing away in one's experience, without approving of some and rejecting other experiences. When one is being Mindful, one is open to all emotions, just as the sun does not choose who or what to shine on.

Mindfulness means seeing how things are, directly and immediately, seeing for oneself that which is present and true. It has the quality of bringing our whole heart and mind, our full attention to each moment. (Goldstein & Kornfield, 1987, p. 62)

Mindfulness is the mind's ability to know what is happening here and now. Emphasize that this knowing is a necessary step in making any change. Mindfulness gives one the space or freedom to "see" what is going on without rushing in to stop, change, or "fix" the experience. Paying attention in this way permits one to "gather the data" of experience and to use this full, mindful awareness as a basis for making decisions about future behavior. Behavior then becomes more skillful, less reactive.

Mindfulness accepts present experience as one of constant change. All experiences arise and pass away like waves on the sea and mindfulness accepts this on a moment-to-moment basis. There is not an attempt to control or fix the present moment or what happens next. (Marlatt, 1994, p. 177)

Many clients with problem eating behaviors spend much of their lives avoiding emotions. Binge eating (and purging) is one method to block emotional awareness; however, emotions become stopped up instead of flowing in and passing away like waves on the sea. Mindfulness, in contrast, involves paying attention to one's emotions, thoughts, physical experiences, and so forth without necessarily trying to terminate or end them. Mindfulness is being open to whatever is happening, accepting and honoring what is happening because it *is* what is happening. It involves learning to be in control of one's own mind by learning how to attend or be aware of one's experiences as fully as possible, learning to be in control of one's attention.

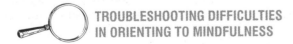

TROUBLESHOOTING DIFFICULTIES IN ORIENTING TO MINDFULNESS

Clients typically have questions or concerns about the practice of Mindfulness. It is important to acknowledge whatever doubts or confusions are raised and address them as best one can. Clients can also be reminded that this is an experiment they can test out. Their task and commitment is to practice these skills during treatment. After wholehearted effort, they can decide at the end of treatment whether or not Mindfulness is useful. Two common questions and possible responses are:

- *Example 1*: "What is the difference between Mindfulness and meditation, or between Mindfulness and hypnosis?"

- *Potential therapist reply*: "Marsha Linehan, who developed dialectical behavior therapy, translated the skills of meditation into behavioral terms. Meditation is often associated with religious connotations, such as meditation as part of Buddhism. *Meditation* is a broader term than *Mindfulness*, and it encompasses a variety of practices for developing your mind in a particular way (e.g., concentration meditation, loving kindness meditation, mindfulness meditation). One purpose might be to develop mindfulness, but people meditate for other reasons as well, such as to develop compassion. Dialectical behavior therapy does not teach meditation. It lays out the concepts and ideas of mindfulness to help you develop your mind to be more aware, clearer seeing, able to access the here and now without judgment, and so forth. In terms of mindfulness versus hypnosis—hypnosis involves focusing awareness, whereas Mindfulness can be either focusing awareness or being aware of multiple events at once."

- *Example 2*: "I've found using a mantra helpful when I practice diaphragmatic breathing rather than just being aware of my breath."

- *Potential therapist reply*: "Some people do notice that focusing the mind on a particular word (e.g., *breathe*) or counting (e.g., from 1 to 10 and then repeating) really helps. It may provide an anchor that helps you become more easily aware of the fact that your mind has wandered."

MINDFULNESS VERSUS BINGE EATING

DISCUSSION POINT: *"Now that we've introduced Mindfulness, do you think you could be Mindful—attending fully to the present moment—and binge (and purge) at the same time?"*

By definition, binge eating involves a loss of control over what one is doing or a lack of awareness about what is going on. Binge eating is frequently a maladaptive means of escaping awareness or blunting experience by not thinking or paying attention to one's emotions or to one's actions. It is an attempt to try to control, change, or get rid of emotions. Mindfulness, on the other hand, is about increasing awareness. Therefore, clients cannot practice Mindfulness *and* binge eat. They are opposite activities. Mindfulness and binge eating are incompatible in the same way that clients cannot be both tense and relaxed. Clients would need to abandon Mindfulness in order to binge eat.

A person cultivates Mindfulness, or the mind's ability to know what is happening, in order to be aware of his or her experience and how his or her mental activities are influencing that experience. For example, usually automatic commentary accompanies a person's experience, and it is frequently evaluative or judgmental. Mindfulness is also being aware of the commentary as just that, commentary and not fact. For example, imagine watching a sports game on television with the volume turned up versus with the sound turned off (i.e., with or without the announcer providing minute-by-minute commentary). The experience would be quite different. Without the commentary, you would simply see just that there is a ball, there is someone who is picking up the ball, and so forth. Compare that with watching the game with all of the excitement and stimulation provided by the commentary in the background. The commentary obviously influences your experience. As another example, you could notice or be mindful of feeling sad and notice the sadness arise and pass away without adding commentary. On the other hand, you could feel sad and add the commentary that "I don't have a good enough reason to feel sad," which might perhaps add guilt or shame to the experience. Mindfulness is paying attention, noticing, and being aware of the sadness and, if present the commentary; it means training the mind not to react to either one but to remain aware of how the mind's commentary or reactivity affects the flow of experience. The point to emphasize is that, by practicing the core Mindfulness skills, clients will be strengthening their ability to know what is happening and to see how their own reactions or inner commentary influences their experience. By recognizing through the use of Mindfulness skills how this process works, one can quiet down the inner commentary and associated emotion dysregulation. Clients might want to experiment with "turning down the volume" to see how different the experience is.

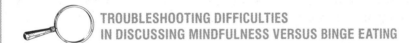

TROUBLESHOOTING DIFFICULTIES IN DISCUSSING MINDFULNESS VERSUS BINGE EATING

Therapists can expect a variety of reactions to the discussion of Mindfulness and binge eating. Such questions and comments can be an opportunity to demonstrate Mindfulness skills. That is, therapists can pay close attention to what is happening and hypothesize about commentary that may be triggering emotional reactions. Therapists can also ask clients to pay careful attention to what they are experiencing and what "commentary" may have prompted the question.

- *Example*: "So many Americans are overweight that it seems unlikely that the whole country is out of touch with their emotions. Isn't the problem in the environment?"

- *Potential therapist reply:* "I want to distinguish between being overweight and binge eating. Not all people who are overweight are binge eaters, and not all binge eaters are overweight. Binge eating is a problem in and of itself that involves not only eating large quantities of food but also feeling a loss of control. The treatment we are undertaking assumes that binge eating results in large part from strong emotions and a deficit of adaptive skills or means to manage these emotions. However, that is not to say that other factors, such as the environment, do not play a role. The key for each of you is to practice and utilize Mindfulness skills to notice and be aware of your own reactions to the environment and how these culminate in binge eating. The same environment does not trigger binge eating in everyone. Developing Mindfulness skills will strengthen your awareness as to how the environment, your emotions, your thoughts, and your behavior lead to binge eating and how to use Mindfulness skills to observe that whole process without reacting with a binge. The treatment model we use to understand binge eating would not necessarily apply to people who are overweight but are not binge eaters."

THE THREE STATES OF MIND:
REASONABLE MIND, EMOTION MIND, AND WISE MIND

The next step in teaching Mindfulness skills is to initiate a discussion about various states of mind. Therapists might ask clients to identify a positive and a negative state of mind and describe the thinking and behaviors that accompany each. The main point to emphasize in this discussion is how one's state of mind influences one's thinking about others, one's view of self, one's behaviors, and so forth. Explain that for the purposes of this treatment, three primary states of mind are identified: Reasonable Mind, Emotion Mind, and Wise Mind. Reasonable Mind is a state of mind in which behaviors are controlled primarily by rationality, whereas Emotion Mind is a state of mind governed primarily by emotions. Wise Mind is the embodiment of Mindfulness skills and synthesizes both Reasonable Mind and Emotion Mind. Yet Wise Mind is not simply adding Reasonable Mind and Emotion Mind together. The quality of Wise Mind is different and is discussed later in this module. Emphasize here that the skills taught in this treatment will enable clients to become more aware of their mind states and to train them to move toward Wise Mind, thereby finding themselves able to make more effective decisions.

Reasonable Mind

Explain that Reasonable Mind is the state of mind in which rational thinking and logic are dominant and therefore primary in determining how clients act. Reason is often what is needed and what is effective for guiding behavior such as balancing checkbooks, solving logical problems, planning and evaluating, and so forth. Reasonable Mind can be very beneficial, but if clients are using reason and logic exclusively to inform behavior and decisions, they might end up overlooking important aspects of a situation or of themselves. Strict reason may be limiting, like monocular as opposed to binocular vision.

An example therapists might use to illustrate this point is that of choosing between two jobs. Imagine that the first job is much more geographically convenient and pays better. The second job pays less and isn't as conveniently located, but it's the one the person is passionate about. Choosing a job based solely on rationality and logic might lead an individual to choose the more convenient and better paying job. However, the person could end up being quite unhappy all day as he or she works at a less satisfying, interesting, or meaningful job. In this scenario, a decision based solely on Reasonable Mind could lead to a decision one regrets. The skills will enable clients to build an awareness of their state of mind so that they will know when they are operating exclusively from Reasonable Mind. Clients would then have the opportunity to access Wise Mind, a state in which they might find the perspective needed to take more effective actions.

DISCUSSION POINT: *"Can you think of examples when Reasonable Mind led to certain decisions? Consider times when such thinking led to beneficial outcomes and when it led to regret."*

Emotion Mind

The other end of the continuum is Emotion Mind. Therapists explain this as the state of mind in which thinking and behavior are governed primarily by the current emotional state, not on the basis of reason. Thinking is hot and emotional rather than cool and rational. "Emotions are regulating you instead of you regulating your emotions." In other words, behaviors such as binge eating (and purging) and other problem behaviors are tightly linked to one's emotions and occur seemingly automatically. By definition, binge eating (and purging) would not occur in Reasonable Mind, in which behavior is based on logic, nor in Wise Mind, in which one is aware and responding on the basis of inner wisdom. When clients are in Emotion Mind and want to act effectively, practicing Mindfulness skills can help them to access Wise Mind and not binge eat (and purge).

Make clear that therapists are not asserting that Emotion Mind does not have a very important place in life. Emotions are powerful motivators of behavior. Clients have only to think of all the accomplishments in the world that were driven by great love or passion. Emotions also provide an invaluable source of information. But when clients' emotions are very hot and intense, the resulting behaviors can be out of touch with clients' core values, such as when they turn to binge eating (and purging). This can set up a cycle in which the problem eating behaviors lead to shame, which, in turn, makes clients more vulnerable to Emotion Mind. Sleep deprivation, stress, illness, and the influence of substances such as alcohol are other examples of things that can increase vulnerability to Emotion Mind, making it more likely that clients would engage in binge eating (and purging).

 DISCUSSION POINT: *"Think of times in your life when only your Emotion Mind was operating. Were there times when this led to behaviors that were helpful to you? Were there times when being governed by your Emotion Mind led to behaviors you regretted? What are some of the factors that make you especially vulnerable to Emotion Mind?"*

Wise Mind

Wise Mind is the state of mind in which clients synthesize all ways of knowing. Aspects of both Reasonable Mind, such as analyzing, and Emotion Mind, such as feelings, are included, but Wise Mind is more than the sum of its parts. For example, Wise Mind includes knowing through intuition, knowing from a place that comes from deep within. It's a state of mind that really taps into one's inner recognition and experiencing of truth. It means knowing something in a very centered way.

Wise Mind has a certain peace; it's not a surface experience. If clients think of Emotion Mind as the waves and ripples on the surface of a pool after a stone has been thrown in, Wise Mind would be the waters underneath. It is that deep, centered place where a person knows something very clearly. Wise Mind is receptive and open. It accepts rather than judges. It is patient rather than impatient. Other terms for Wise Mind are *true self, spirit, consciousness*, or *heart of hearts*.

In Wise Mind, the client's best self takes over. Action is effective when its basis is wise knowing. In fact, a wise response may be to *not act at all* but to just maintain awareness of the urge to act—for example, being aware of urges to binge but not acting on these urges. Wise Mind is aware of emotions and reason as they come and go but is not controlled by them. The therapist's self-disclosure about his or her use of Wise Mind in everyday life can be especially effective in illustrating the concept. As an example, one of our therapists disclosed the following:

"I have worked a great deal to figure out what it is that I'm really feeling inside. I've had to have a strong intention to separate myself and what I think from absorbing what someone else around me thinks. For example, I have a significant other who is the kind of driver who always believes there's sufficient time to make a turn against an oncoming driver. I am a more cautious driver. One day we were driving and as usual my partner was pressing me to just go ahead and take the turn. In a gut way I knew that this was not the time to press my luck because it was a busy intersection at rush hour, and, in fact, just then a car rushed by. This was the right decision for me and involved trusting my own sense and not doing something to please my partner. That's an example of Wise Mind in my everyday life. I know I've been able to tune into it when it feels like a gut response from deep within. I don't want to make it sound like Wise Mind is necessarily calm. Imagine making a decision about separating conjoint twins. You would use all the current science to make a Wise Mind decision. Though you might find a level of peace with the decision, it wouldn't be calm. It would be agonizing. The point is that you would know you had made a Wise Mind decision even when it might be the most difficult and wrenching decision you've ever had to make."

 DISCUSSION POINT: *"Take a minute to think of a time in your life when your behavior was influenced by your access to your Wise Mind."*

It is useful to point out that *everyone* has a Wise Mind—whether or not it has ever been experienced: Having a Wise Mind is like having a heart. It is part of the definition of being a human being and everybody has one. However, some hearts are stronger than others, and this can be influenced by the amount of exercise one does, the amount of attention one pays to strengthening this muscle. Binge eating (and purging), mindless eating, and other problematic eating behaviors interfere with being in touch with Wise Mind—with one's best self, with one's clarity of being, with that clear inner sense of what's important. Especially initially, clients may not have ready access to their Wise Minds or may not have experienced this connection lately.

Therapists may wish to use the next exercise to offer clients a chance to practice accessing Wise Mind and to be helped to avoid acting on urges to use food. It is important to make clear that no one client's experience of Wise Mind will be the same as anyone else's. Furthermore, there is no formula or set of tricks to accessing Wise Mind. Clients will have to determine which ways work best for them; the following exercise is just one option. Clarify that although one cannot force access, this does not mean that one cannot do anything to better position oneself for such access. Practicing the Mindfulness skills, for example, paves the way or sets up the conditions for accessing Wise Mind. It brings one "into the vicinity." The following script can be modified as needed.

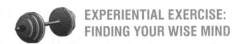

EXPERIENTIAL EXERCISE: FINDING YOUR WISE MIND

"Let's start off finding a place for your eyes to gently focus so that you're not distracted. Let the chair fully support you as you sit comfortably, your legs on the floor and your hands on your knees or lap. Imagine a string is running through your head up to the ceiling, keeping you upright. If you find your mind wandering, notice this and bring it gently back to the exercise. We'll begin by following your breath. This is often a helpful way to facilitate mindfulness, as it anchors you into the present moment. You don't have to do any type of special breathing, just be aware of your breathing. It may help to initially note the sensation of air moving in and out of your nostrils. And as you breathe, see if you can go into yourself and find a place of calmness, of peace. Some people find it helpful to imagine themselves as a stone or pebble slowly sinking into a warm lake. The surface of the lake has ripples, but as you sink down into the water, it becomes more still. Imagine yourself floating down ... gently ... slowly. Allow yourself to sink and settle calmly into the sandy bottom of the lake. You are at rest. The sandy bottom is fully supporting you. From this quiet, peaceful place, you have distance from the choppy surface, and you can get in touch with your core values. Operating from your Wise Mind, you can see and respond to what is, to reality. You are your true self, your spirit, your consciousness. You become open to experience itself. Let your deep inner wisdom give you direction in guiding your actions so that they're consistent with your values. Now, take three deep, slow, flowing breaths as you leave this image."

DISCUSSION POINT:
"What was that experience like for you?"

Therapists emphasize that the most important thing about learning to use the skill of accessing Wise Mind is to practice, practice, practice! Because clients are most vulnerable to binge eating (and purging) when in Emotion Mind, they might find it helpful to try to notice when emotions are beginning to become very intense. The goal is for clients to reach the point at which they wake up to the fact that their actions are being controlled by their Emotion Mind. This awareness in and of itself helps to break the automatic link between emotional dysregulation and problematic eating behaviors. By then focusing on their breathing and anchoring in the present, clients should gradually find themselves more and more skillful at shifting from Emotion Mind to their inner wisdom.

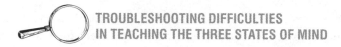

TROUBLESHOOTING DIFFICULTIES IN TEACHING THE THREE STATES OF MIND

- *Example*: "Does binge eating always take place in Emotion Mind, when you're triggered by emotions? It seems as much a habit as anything else."

- *Potential therapist reply*: "It's important to be clear about how one defines 'habit.' Some people use the word to imply that something just happens—that it takes place without a cue and cannot necessarily be understood. To my way of thinking, binge eating is a learned behavior. What I definitely believe, however, is that over time it can become so 'overlearned' that it starts to feel automatic. That's why it's so helpful to use the chain analysis. When I think of a 'habit,' I think of a lack of awareness. That lack of awareness is not Wise Mind. Without the awareness, one couldn't be in touch with which emotions one was experiencing. Binge eating is also not effective behavior and so would probably not be Wise Mind behavior. By gaining access to a wise, peaceful state of mind, your experience of what now feels like a 'habit' may broaden."

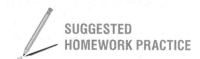

SUGGESTED HOMEWORK PRACTICE

1. Therapists instruct clients to complete the Wise Mind Homework Sheet (Appendix 4.2). Clients should write about an experience in which they use their Wise Mind over the following week. Clients should pay attention to a time when they noticed that their thoughts and behaviors were driven by their Emotion Mind and felt an urge to engage in problem eating behavior. At that time they should practice accessing their Wise Mind by asking "What would my Wise Mind say here?" or "How would I respond wisely?"

2. Therapists instruct clients to fill out the Emotion Mind and Reasonable Mind Homework Sheets (Appendices 4.3 and 4.4), writing about at least one instance of being in each state of mind during the following week. In particular, clients should notice what gets them into Emotion Mind and how this state of mind differs from Wise Mind and Reasonable Mind. Therapists should point out that by using these writing exercises, clients will increase their awareness of what state of mind they are in.

3. Therapists suggest that clients make it a point to practice getting in touch with their Wise Minds every day. Purposely setting aside time to practice will be most helpful, so as not to become distracted by trying to do something else simultaneously. Therapists encourage clients by reminding them that it may take a while to find their Wise Minds and that a helpful way to practice is to begin by using diaphragmatic breathing, bringing their attention to their breath. Once clients have found their Wise Minds, they will often find it a good time to renew their commitment to refrain from binge eating (and purging) and other problem eating behaviors.

ORIENTATION TO MINDFULNESS "WHAT" SKILLS

The core Mindfulness skills include two sets of skills to help strengthen the client's ability to open her or his Wise Mind. The first set of these includes the "What" skills. They answer the question *"What* do individuals do to try to facilitate getting in touch with their Wise Minds?" These skills are Observe, Describe, and Participate.

Observe

The skill Observe involves sensing or experiencing without labeling or putting words to the experience. In other words, clients are placing attention on something and noticing the experience without getting caught up in it, judging it, or reacting to it. Like a guard watching over a castle gate, clients will use Observe to control where they place attention but not what they see. Point out that clients can use Observe for things that are outside themselves, or they can step inside and Observe their internal experiences—such as their thoughts and/or emotions. Remind clients that it is much harder to engage in binge eating (and purging) or other problem behaviors when they are focused on observing urges to binge or the sensations of eating. As therapists make clear, it is necessary to be able to step back and Observe in order to have a wise and nonreactive awareness of events. Therapists may wish to use the following sample script, modifying as needed, to experientially introduce the skill.

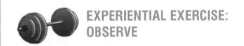 **EXPERIENTIAL EXERCISE:**
OBSERVE

"Put both feet on the floor. Place your awareness on your feet and just observe the experience of your feet on the floor. It's stepping back from an experience without words. You aren't describing the experience of your feet on the floor; you are just placing your attention there. You can notice the experience without anything else, without words or judgment. Just observe. It's a bare-bones awareness. Now place your awareness on the muscles in your neck and shoulders. Just observe the experience, the sensation in your neck and shoulders, without words. Just let your attention be there—stepping back from the experience, just being aware of it."

Observing means allowing oneself to experience awareness in the moment, *whatever* is happening. Observing an experience does not mean trying to change it, to put words on it, nor to terminate it. When clients are practicing Observe, they are stepping back, letting their experiences be there. They are holding their experiences but not adding anything more.

Therapists inform clients that this observing stance may be applied toward emotional experiencing. For example, if a client wants to practice observing sadness, this would mean allowing the sadness to be there as part of the moment without trying to change it, make it different, or run from it. Clients may practice observing with any emotion, whether it be anger, anxiety, joy, or other. If clients do not know what emotion it is they are observing, they might try to observe accompanying physical sensations, such as shallow breathing, clammy hands, a pounding heart, or the sensation of one's face reddening.

Observing requires the ability to step back and observe in a nonattached way. It is important that clients understand that observing can be separated from the response itself. Therapists describe how a person's heart beating and *observing* one's heart beating are separate phenomena. The person's heart is beating all the time, whether he or she observes it or not. *Observing* it beat is a different response from the heart beating. Similarly, clients may observe their thinking, which is different from the response of thinking itself. Therapists underscore that this holds true with emotions—clients can observe or watch emotions, which is different from experiencing the emotions themselves. Indeed, clients may have many emotions going on that they may or may not be aware of, emotions that they are not really observing.

Therapists might use the helpful analogy of how observing is similar to being in the eye of a hurricane, with the client's life unfolding and emotions potentially "swirling" all around. With Observe, there is a calm center into which clients can step back to watch and maintain awareness of what is swirling around without getting caught up in it. Clients do not get swept away but just Observe.

Suggest that clients begin practicing observing physical sensations before moving to observing larger, more complicated phenomena, such as emotions. A way for clients to strengthen their ability to Observe is to practice observing their feet on the floor, hands on a table, the physical sensations of facial muscles, the sounds surrounding them while sitting, and so forth.

Describe

Describe, the second "What" skill, involves using words to represent what it is that clients observe. When practicing Describe, clients label a thought as a thought ("I'm noticing the thought, 'This is hard'"), a feeling as a feeling ("I'm experiencing the feeling of frustration"), and/or a sensation as a sensation ("My hands are cold"). Therapists emphasize that when practicing Describe, clients are not adding a judgment to the description (e.g., "It's bad to have that thought or this emotion"). Describe means not adding a moral dimension to one's experience but just putting words to the experience as it is.

Make sure that clients understand the potential difference between a thought and a fact. For example, if a client notices the thought " Two plus two equals four," his or her thought, in this case, is a fact. Too often clients aren't thinking about facts, yet they treat their thoughts as facts. For example, take the thought, "I'm no good." A client might treat this thought as if it were a fact. As therapists should clarify, practicing the skill of Describe in this case would involve saying, "I just had the thought 'I'm no good.'" Therapists make sure clients appreciate the distinction between labeling "I'm no good" as a thought and making the thought sound like a fact by saying to oneself, "I'm no good." The former involves being able to observe what is going on in one's mind and then describing it. Therapists may wish to use the following script, modifying as needed, when introducing the conveyer belt exercise, an experiential exercise that involves the Observe and Describe skills.

EXPERIENTIAL EXERCISE:
OBSERVE AND DESCRIBE WITH A "CONVEYER BELT"

"First, sit in your chair with your feet on the floor, imagining a string from your head to the ceiling, with your back similarly aligned. Find a place for your eyes to look that won't distract you. Here is an exercise that I find useful when I'm in a situation that I can't control—such as being stuck in traffic and feeling very anxious about being late for a meeting. [Note: A self-disclosure involving the therapist's experience of actually practicing the skill to be taught is an effective way of introducing it. Therapists should feel free to substitute a different self-disclosure here.]

"I find this exercise very helpful to reduce my emotion's intensity. You might find it helpful when your emotions start getting intense and you're feeling an urge to engage in binge eating and/or purging. Take several deep breaths. ... Imagine that your experience is on a conveyer belt. You can think of it as your stream of consciousness. Basically, your thoughts, your feelings, your sensations, your impulses, your action urges—all of these are coming down a conveyer belt that is passing in front of you. You are stepping back within yourself and just noticing, you are just watching what is coming down the conveyer belt. First you observe and then you describe, you put words on what you see. For example, 'Here's a memory, here's a tingling sensation, here's a hollow sensation in my stomach, a feeling of guilt, an urge to scratch an itch, an urge to eat. ...' Just let it be whatever it is. You're noticing without reacting. It's just a moment-to-moment experience of describing, with words, what you observe on the conveyer belt. Don't try to stop the conveyer belt should you notice something you particularly like on it or attempt to push things off that you dislike. Just step back within yourself, observing and describing. ... Take three deep diaphragmatic breaths before ending the exercise."

Explain that Observe and Describe are very effective skills for clients to use when they feel their Emotion Minds are getting ramped up. For example, if clients feels themselves beginning to have an urge to binge eat and/or purge or engage in other problematic eating behaviors, they can practice stepping back, taking a breath, and simply observing their feet on the floor. Or clients may put their experience on the conveyer belt. Therapists point out that when clients observe and then describe their experience with words, they are slowing that experience down. Wise Mind can be used to help clients know when to move ahead.

Participate

Therapists introduce Participate, the last "What" skill, by explaining that this skill involves entering fully into one's experience, being fully aware, fully attending. When participating, clients are in their experience, having direct contact with it, and letting go of self-consciousness. Therapists might suggest that clients imagine the process of learning a dance step. At first one would observe others doing the sequence of steps. Then one would describe what is observed, such as "step to the right, pause, step to the left." Finally, once one knows the steps, the point is reached at which one is immersed in the moment, becoming "one" with the activity. The goal of the "What" skills is to be able to participate.

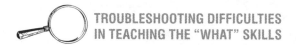

TROUBLESHOOTING DIFFICULTIES IN TEACHING THE "WHAT" SKILLS

- *Example 1*: "I get so caught up in things that I can't step back and detach enough to Observe or Describe."

- *Potential therapist reply*: "What you would Observe and Describe would be exactly that! For example, you might say, 'I notice I'm getting caught up in my experience and having a hard time separating.' That's part of the experience. There's no way to do this 'wrong,' because it's all your experience. What I think is happening is that you're judging as you Observe and Describe. So again, that's part of the experience. 'I'm noticing the judgment. I'm not doing this right.' Just put it all on the conveyer belt."

- *Example 2*: "It's easier for me to observe my feet on the floor without judging than to observe other parts of my body, like my shoulders."

- *Potential therapist reply*: "To strengthen your skill with the essence of Observe, practice observing things that are easier and less complicated first. It sounds like practicing observing your feet on the floor is the kind of exercise you should be doing now so that you can build up your skill."

- *Example 3*: "I can't seem to be able to observe without describing."

- *Potential therapist reply*: "Observing without describing is sensing. If you're describing at the same time as you observe, just notice the describing. Many people have the same difficulty at first. You'll be able to separate them over time with continued practice."

- *Example 4*: "It seems like with Observe and Wise Mind that I'm stepping back from my emotion. Is there a time to just feel my emotions, or should I try not to have my emotions because they might lead me to binge eat [and purge]?"

- *Potential therapist reply*: "The idea is not to avoid emotions or emotional experiences, but to be aware of them. In Emotion Mind, people often aren't paying attention or aware of their emotions because they're reacting to them. They're binge eating or doing other things to avoid feeling or to distract themselves in an attempt to get rid of an emotion. So the goal is to be aware of your feelings without reacting to them with actions or behaviors."

- *Example 5*: "It seems like a lot of the skills overlap."

- *Potential therapist reply*: "In a sense they do, or at least your practice of them can. For example, you could start out practicing diaphragmatic breathing, then practice Observe and Describe, and end up in Wise Mind."

Mindful Eating

Mindful Eating, the next Mindfulness skill, is participating fully in each moment with full awareness that one is eating. When clients eat mindfully, they are using their "What" skills of Observe, Describe, and Participate. It is helpful to make clear that, by definition, participation involves Wise Mind and full awareness. Binge eating may feel like participating because clients become very involved in the act of eating. But binge eating by definition is mindless because there is no effective awareness of the consequences of one's behavior. Nothing exists except the food. Clients are on autopilot and are shutting down awareness. Like binge eating, mindless eating also involves unawareness.

In our research studies, we have found it helpful to use an experiential exercise to teach Mindful Eating. Based on work by Kabat-Zinn (1990), we use raisins. Therapists may wish to choose other foods for this exercise, either as substitutes or in addition (e.g., chocolate chips). The following script may be useful, modifying as needed.

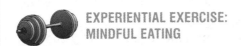 **EXPERIENTIAL EXERCISE:
MINDFUL EATING**

"For this exercise, we are practicing Mindfulness with a Mindful Eating exercise. This particular exercise comes from a book called *Full Catastrophe Living* by Jon Kabat-Zinn [1990]. He has used Mindfulness as a basis for a stress-reduction program he started at the University of Massachusetts Medical Center. These Mindfulness skills were found to be effective for reducing pain in individuals suffering from chronic pain syndromes.

"Please take three raisins and hold them in your hand. Begin by observing them in your palm, bringing your attention to each raisin. Observe each individual raisin carefully, as if you had never seen a raisin before. You might imagine that you're like a Martian, seeing a raisin for the first time. Really take the time to observe. For example, notice the different shapes, surfaces, and colors. Notice the texture with your fingers. While you are observing, be aware of any thoughts that come into your mind about raisins or eating raisins. Now, bring just one raisin to your nose and smell. Fully know what the smell of one raisin is like, have full awareness of it. Now, with awareness of your arm and hand moving, place the raisin in your mouth. Be aware of your mouth, your tongue. Then, very slowly, experience the taste of one raisin by chewing it very slowly. Notice the texture on your tongue, on the roof of your mouth. Notice how the raisin feels as you bite into it with your teeth. Notice any impulses to swallow the raisin. Then, when you are ready, swallow it—following the taste as long as you can as it goes down your throat. Observe, Describe, and Participate fully in the experience of eating just this one raisin.

"Eat each of the raisins in this way, chewing each one slowly, really tasting it, noticing where the raisin is in your mouth, listening to the sounds of the chewing, being fully aware. Notice whether there are any differences between the first raisin and the others. Does the taste change after you have already eaten one? Notice your experience with each chew. You are mindfully eating—putting all your attention and awareness on this one thing you are doing. You are literally more awake, rather than on the autopilot of mechanically eating without full awareness. When you participate, you are attending to eating. So you really taste this one raisin. You have the experience."

Therapists emphasize that Mindful Eating involves all three of the "What" skills. First, clients cannot describe something unless they first observe it. Then, while eating, clients are participating. Clients are not on autopilot or eating raisins "hand to mouth." They are eating with full awareness and attention to the experience of eating.

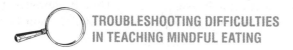 **DISCUSSION POINT:** *"What was your experience? Is this how you normally eat things? If not, how is it different? How can you use this experience to prevent binge eating (and purging)?"*

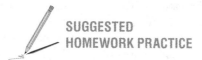 ## TROUBLESHOOTING DIFFICULTIES IN TEACHING MINDFUL EATING

• *Example*: "It's impossible to mindfully eat in our everyday lives the way we ate the raisin."

• *Potential therapist reply*: "It may not be possible to eat exactly the way we practiced Mindful Eating all of the time. That exercise was meant to give you an idea of how to practice the skill. A rehearsal for a play may not be exactly the same experience as when you perform it. If you are with others at a restaurant, your use of Mindful Eating would probably be different. But that doesn't mean that the breadbasket would be emptied without your noticing. You might eat a few bites mindfully, then participate in the conversation, then eat a few more bites. It may not be that you're eating exactly the way you ate the raisins. But it would be a different experience, certainly, from eating mindlessly."

SUGGESTED HOMEWORK PRACTICE

1. Therapists instruct clients to fill out the Mindfulness "What" Skills Homework Sheet (Appendix 4.5).

2. Therapists instruct clients to practice Mindful Eating on at least three occasions over the following week or until the next session, writing about their practice on the "What" Skills Homework Sheet (Appendix 4.5).

ORIENTATION TO "HOW" SKILLS

Introduce the Mindfulness "How" skills as answering the question *"How* do you practice the 'What' skills of Observe, Describe, and Participate to access Wise Mind?" These "How" skills include Nonjudgmentally, One-Mindfully, and Effectively.

Nonjudgmentally

The first "How" skill involves taking a nonjudgmental stance when Observing, Describing, and Participating. In other words, this skill means that one is not evaluating something or someone as good or bad, right or wrong, valuable or not, worthwhile or worthless. The aim is to describe in terms of consequences. For example, clients may Observe and Describe the consequences of binge eating (and purging) in terms of the harmful effects on their self-esteem and physical health. They may also Observe and Describe the fact that they want to change their problematic eating behaviors. *Nonjudgmentally* means not adding the judgment that one is a *bad* person for binge eating (and purging) or a *good* person for not doing so.

As therapists remind them, clients are not stopping binge eating (and purging) for moral reasons. Clients are stopping because they've *Observed* and *Described* that binge eating (and purging) is destructive—making them feel sick; wasting time, energy, and money; and inevitably leading them to feel miserable. The point here, therapists emphasize, is for clients to stop getting stuck in the good–bad, right–wrong dichotomy of judging and, instead, to notice consequences.

Therapists might provide examples of common judgments: "I'm a failure," "I'm no good," or "I'm stupid." It is helpful for therapists to highlight how insidious judgmental thinking can be. Many clients are often not even aware that they are judging. Therapists underscore how judgments have a profound effect on emotions and behavior. Therapists might suggest that when clients find themselves feeling depressed "for no particular reason," they may not be aware of how these emotions were triggered by a bout of self-judging.

Therapists describe how practicing the skill of being Nonjudgmental involves cultivating a nonjudgmental attitude toward one's experience and what comes up in one's mind. Practicing Nonjudgmentally also means increasing awareness of the amount of judging that takes place. Acknowledge that dropping judging is difficult, and make clear how important it is that, when clients become aware of a tendency to judge, they not treat themselves judgmentally! Instead, the goal is to simply Observe and Describe their judgments, not judge their judging. Remind clients of the conveyer belt exercise, in which clients may practice the Nonjudgmental stance. For example, clients might notice a judgment coming down the conveyer belt. At that point, clients can Observe and Describe its presence. Perhaps, especially if the judgments are frequent, clients might almost want to "wave" at the judgment, acknowledging that "Yes, there's that judgment about the shape of my body again" or "Yes, there's that judgment I have about the fact that I have an eating disorder in the first place."

Therapists illustrate the distinction between judging and noticing consequences by inviting clients to think about the different effect of saying "I am a bad parent because I snapped at my child" versus saying "My snapping at my child hurt his feelings, which I don't want to do and would like to work to change." The first sentence is a judgment, whereas the second one emphasizes the consequences.

 DISCUSSION POINT:
"Does the skill of Nonjudgmentally seem relevant to you?"

Often judgments masquerade as facts. For example, the statement "I am overweight" may be a fact, but if the judgment "Being overweight is bad and overweight people are less worthy than normal weight or thin people" is implied, then the judging piggybacks on the statement of fact and gets mistaken for part of the fact.

 DISCUSSION POINT: *"Can you think of any examples of your judgments masquerading as facts?"*

Judgments are not preferences, values, or emotions. For example, the statement "I like jazz better than country music" is a preference, not a judgment. Judgments such as "this is better than this" can have their place in providing feedback (e.g., grades) or information to a person about what to continue, change, or stop. The problem is not so much with this type of judging that provides information. The difficulty arises when the judgment is presented as a statement of fact, such as saying that jazz is *better* than country music.

Point out that negative self-judging is similar to self-invalidation. As we discussed during the description of the consequences of the invalidating environment, many clients with a history of engaging in problematic eating behaviors have difficulty validating themselves. They seem to invalidate themselves automatically or, in other words, mindlessly—without awareness. Self-invalidation and negative self-judging can be thought of as stomping all over one's experience, including feelings, thoughts, and actions. For example, clients may or may not be aware of how often they judge themselves as failures. Such a judgment, however, may be the trigger for an emotion such as despondency or depression. This may start them on the path to binge eating (and purging) as a maladaptive means of escaping from the negative emotions triggered by inner judging. Instead, observing the contents of one's mind, labeling a judgment as a judgment, and letting it go down the conveyer belt brings awareness to the otherwise automatic link between self-judging and its consequences.

⊚ **DISCUSSION POINT:** *"Take a moment and ask yourself how judging operates in your life. Does it play a role in your internal chain of events leading to binge eating and/or purging? How key a role do you think it plays?"*

One-Mindfully

The second "How" skill, One-Mindfully, involves learning to control one's attention. With One-Mindfully, the mind focuses on just one thing at a time, one moment at a time. Attention is not divided. Clients are fully present in just this one moment. Impatience involves tapping one's foot, wanting to get out of this present moment, and wanting to move on. In contrast, when practicing patience, clients are letting things be as they are in the moment, One-Mindfully. Thus, when thinking about One-Mindfully, remember patience and letting go.

One-Mindfully brings the whole of one's person to bear on the present activity, whether it be eating, driving, listening, or thinking about a problem, without letting attention wander to something else. One-Mindfully also involves becoming aware of when one's mind wanders and controlling attention to bring it back to the present moment and the present activity, no matter what it is.

For example, when clients are brushing their teeth, practicing One-Mindfully means just brushing their teeth. One-Mindfully is related to concentration, being able to stay focused. The idea is to try to stay in the moment, even if only for some moments of one's life. By anticipating the future or ruminating over the past, clients miss out on what is happening in the present, in this moment. Make the point that life is only a series of moments.

The following experiential exercise is an opportunity to practice Mindful Eating with a typical binge food. Clients first practice this imaginally. The skill of One-Mindfully is being highlighted, but the skills of Observe, Describe, and Participate (at least imaginally) are also being practiced. The script can be modified as needed.

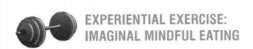

EXPERIENTIAL EXERCISE:
IMAGINAL MINDFUL EATING

"Begin by finding a place for your eyes to softly focus that won't distract you. Let the chair fully support you, with your feet on the floor and your head aligned as if a string were attached from it to the ceiling. Take several deep, flowing breaths and bring to mind a food that you might typically binge on, if you have a typical food. Perhaps pizza, ice cream, chips, or whatever. Bring your full attention, your undivided attention, to just this food, as we did with the raisins. Smell the food, look at it, observe its colors. Take one chew at a time, experience one flavor at a time, with your full attention on the act of eating, on chewing. If your mind wanders, just bring it back to the activity you're engaged in, just eating. Stay with the eating, one small swallow at a time. You might be aware of thoughts that this doesn't taste good or, as many of you described when you practiced mindful eating, that you didn't really want it. But the point is to have a full awareness of eating."

 DISCUSSION POINT: *"What was your imaginary Mindful Eating like? Are you willing to eat this way in reality?"*

Effectively

Introduce the last "How" skill, Effectively, by explaining that this skill involves focusing on doing what works, on being effective. Therapists make clear that being right, being correct, or being perfect are not the issue. The idea is to do what is effective to achieve one's goal. Effectively means playing with the cards you are dealt rather than folding. Effectively means playing by the rules, even if clients do not like the rules or are afraid of them. Practicing being effective is the absolute opposite of cutting off your nose to spite your face.

Therapists bring up how, at times, practicing Effectively means that one has to give in instead of insisting that things go the way one wants them. Indeed, insisting that things go a certain way, that that is the only right way, is a kind of digging in that can often propel one into Emotion Mind and into binge eating and/or purging and other problem eating behaviors. Clients *may* be right; the client's way might indeed *be* the fair way. But when clients rigidly adhere to something that isn't in line with the present reality, things just will not work. Being effective requires accepting reality as it is and acknowledging the situation as it is, not the situation the way clients think it should be. Things are not always fair.

Therapists might use the example of imagining what would happen if a client visits a busy city and decides that because people *should* be trustworthy, one *should not* have to lock one's car and *should* be able to leave packages inside it while going for a walk in a nearby park. If one's goal is to eventually take one's purchases home, would this likely be an effective action?

Effectively means focusing on what one's goals are, such as wanting to enjoy one's purchases or wanting to stop binge eating (and purging) and other problematic eating behaviors. Clients are thinking about what is effective rather than insisting that the world or their bodies be different from what they are. This includes letting go of binge eating (and purging), because this behavior is not effective. Instead, what *is* effective is getting in touch with one's Wise Mind and being mindful of consequences.

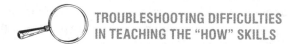 **DISCUSSION POINT:** *"Can you think of a time when you were shooting yourself in the foot in some way and that escalated your emotions and led to binge eating and/or purging?"*

TROUBLESHOOTING DIFFICULTIES IN TEACHING THE "HOW" SKILLS

- *Example 1*: "I'm too busy not to multitask!"

- *Potential therapist reply*: "I can so relate to that! You have to use your Wise Mind. I'm not saying that change is easy. It could feel excruciating at times. But if you're going to be different, change is required."

- *Example 2*: "Doing things One-Mindfully sounds so difficult!"

- *Potential therapist reply*: "People describe a lot of different experiences when practicing the skill of One-Mindfully. People often worry that if they experience an emotion One-Mindfully, then that means the experience will never change. For example, if they're experiencing fear, then they'll be stuck in the fear forever. But it is the nature of experience that experience changes."

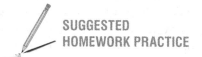 ### SUGGESTED HOMEWORK PRACTICE

Therapists instruct clients to complete the Mindfulness "How" Skills Homework Sheet (Appendix 4.6).

Urge Surfing

Therapists introduce this skill by explaining that Urge Surfing uses the Mindfulness skills of Observe and Describe to "surf" out urges to binge (and purge), preoccupations with food, and cravings. Mindful Urge Surfing involves a mindful nonattached observing of these urges. With this skill, clients are learning to accept the urges, cravings, and preoccupations without reacting to them, judging them, or, particularly, acting on them. Clients can simply observe and describe the ebb and flow of their urges. They are detaching the urge from the object of the urge—the food. Instead of engaging in eating the food and/or purging it, they are to practice observing and describing their urges.

Make clear that the idea is for clients to use Urge Surfing to train their brains not to respond to urges, as they had done previously. In other words, when they gave in to their urges and binged or engaged in other problematic eating behaviors, they reinforced the link between having an urge and acting on it. Urge Surfing involves retraining their brain. Over time, by Urge Surfing urges, cravings, and preoccupations, the brain learns that it is possible to experience an urge without acting on it. Therapists explain that clients may find it helpful to think of Urge Surfing as being similar to surfing or riding out a wave. The wave is the urge. Instead of trying to stop its movement, clients can surf on top of it. In doing so, clients are using the skills of Observe and Describe to stay with the experience without succumbing to it. Clients should notice the urge moment by moment, particularly how, like a wave, it evolves and shifts over time. The key to Urge Surfing is the stepping back and not reacting. The following experiential exercise allows clients to practice Urge Surfing with a food that many find tempting. Modify the script as needed. Begin this exercise by handing out malt balls (or other type of tempting candy).

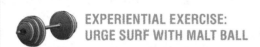

EXPERIENTIAL EXERCISE: URGE SURF WITH MALT BALL

"Take one of the malt balls but do not eat it. First, look at the malt ball, or, alternatively, imagine some other food you find more tempting. Smell it, be aware of any salivation. Be mindful of any thoughts, feelings, or judgments that arise. Be very aware of any urges to eat the malt ball. Again, the idea is to stay with the urges without eating. Just be open to whatever comes to mind. Just urge surf, riding the urge out. Use Observe, Describe, Nonjudgmentally, and One-Mindfully with all that you experience—any thoughts, sensations, feelings, or judgments you experience as you are aware of the malt ball. You may want to visualize the malt ball as though it were a picture of a malt ball instead of the actual food in front of you. Imagining food as a picture of the food can be helpful to separate yourself from it. You are not reacting to the urge. At the end of this exercise, get in touch with your Wise Mind to decide whether to eat the malt ball or not. If you choose to eat it, do so as a conscious choice to eat it—and do so mindfully. If you choose not to eat it, be mindful of that choice."

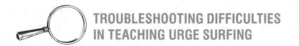

TROUBLESHOOTING DIFFICULTIES IN TEACHING URGE SURFING

- *Example*: "With Urge Surfing, are you saying we're on the waves or somewhere else—observing them?"
- *Potential therapist reply*: "The image of a wave is a metaphor for the experience one has when one is caught up in one's emotion and is noticing a strong pull to act in a way that is consistent with that emotion. You're imagining that you are surfing the urge as if it were a wave. You're watching it rise higher and higher, and then start to fall. It may seem as if it never stops rising, but it *will* always fall. In a sense, in order to surf, you do have to be riding your board on top of the wave while at the same time observing your stance with respect to the wave. But I suppose you could also step back and watch yourself Urge Surfing the waves."

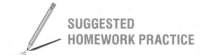

Therapists instruct clients to fill out the Urge Surfing Homework Sheet describing their practice of this skill over the following week or until the next session (Appendix 4.7).

Alternate Rebellion

Introduce this skill by explaining that many clients with eating disorders describe their binge eating as a wish to rebel or "get back" at those who have been judgmental about their weight and/or eating—such as friends, family members, and society in general. Alternate Rebellion is the skill of satisfying this wish to rebel without destroying the client's overriding objective, which is to stop binge eating (and purging). Alternate Rebellion involves rebelling Effectively. As the therapist describes, it involves finding a way to honor the urge to rebel creatively instead of attempting to suppress or judge it or to mindlessly give into it by binge eating or other problematic eating behaviors.

Therapists may find it helpful to elicit reasons that binge eating (and purging) is not an effective strategy for rebelling in that clients' overall objectives for obtaining a higher quality of life are not kept in mind. With Alternate Rebellion, the idea is to try to figure out how to satisfy the urge to rebel in a manner that honors it and the client. Alternate Rebellion can also replace the target behavior of capitulating—of shutting down the option to not binge (and purge). Make clear that there are many ways to employ this skill, and invite clients to use their imagination. For example, clients who feel very judged by others about what they eat might effectively rebel by going to an ice cream store, ordering one cone, and eating it mindfully, without hiding, rather than buying a pint at a grocery store and eating it secretively at home. Some clients describe effectively practicing Alternate Rebellion by buying sexy lingerie that flaunts and celebrates their bodies exactly as they are. Others have practiced Alternate Rebellion by writing a letter to someone that says every single thing they want to say with no censoring—then burning the letter.

Therapists might point out that many clients with eating disorders give themselves a list of rules about how they must look or what they must eat and then find themselves acting as if those rules were actually someone else's. In such cases, clients are really rebelling against their own rules. An Alternate Rebellion, in such cases, might be to let go of overly rigid rules. If a client is exhausting him- or herself by insisting that project after project be completed, for example, an effective Alternate Rebellion might be to sleep in! The key is to use Wise Mind. In some cases, Wise Mind might say that another skill might be more effective for experiencing the urge to rebel rather than acting on it. But if Wise Mind decides to honor the rebellion, then the key is for the client to act in such a way that they will not harm themselves.

DISCUSSION POINT: *"What comes to mind regarding how you might satisfy and honor the wish to rebel without destroying your overall goal of stopping binge eating and/or purging?"*

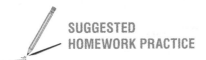

SUGGESTED
HOMEWORK PRACTICE

Therapists instruct clients to fill out the Alternate Rebellion Homework Sheet (Appendix 4.8) describing their practice of this skill over the following week or until the next session.

List of Mindfulness Core Skills

- Wise Mind
- Observe ⎫
- Describe ⎬ Mindfulness "What" Skills
- Participate ⎭
- Mindful Eating
- Nonjudgmentally ⎫
- One-Mindfully ⎬ Mindfulness "How" Skills
- Effectively ⎭
- Urge Surfing
- Alternate Rebellion

APPENDIX 4.2

Wise Mind Homework Sheet

Wise Mind is intuitive, calm, peaceful, and sure. Wise Mind is an integration of all ways of knowing: by observing, feeling, analyzing, intuition, and so forth. In Wise Mind, there is a sense of knowing, of understanding, of experiencing truth. It involves knowing something in a very centered way. Wise Mind is an experience that comes from deep within, not from your current emotional state. Wise Mind means that your best self, your wise self, guides you. In Wise Mind your true self and values, your own internal wisdom, guide you.

Instructions: In the following space and on the back of this sheet, write about your experiences of (1) finding your Wise Mind, (2) experiencing your Wise Mind, and (3) asking yourself, "What does my Wise Mind say?" Describe what you did to find your Wise Mind. Describe your experience of your Wise Mind. Practice asking yourself, "What would my Wise Mind say?" and "What is wise responding?" when an Emotion Mind behavior threatens and urges to binge, purge, and/or eat mindlessly arise. Describe on this practice sheet what your Wise Mind says.

Emotion Mind Homework Sheet

Emotion Mind means that your emotions are in control—that your thinking and actions are controlled by your current emotional state. Thinking is hot rather than cool and rational. Behavior is reactive and lightning fast, rather than measured and with consequences logically considered.

Instructions: Describe in the following space times during the week when your Emotion Mind was in control. Describe the circumstances that evoked your Emotion Mind, as well as your Emotion Mind thinking, actions, and sensations. Describe your experience of Emotion Mind, as well as the consequences or outcome of your Emotion Mind taking control. What would have been different had your Wise Mind been in control?

Reasonable Mind Homework Sheet

Reasonable Mind means that rational thinking and logic are in control of what you do. In Reasonable Mind, thinking and emotions are cool, and situations are approached in a measured and nonreactive manner.

Instructions: Describe times during the week when your Reasonable Mind was in control. Describe the circumstances that evoked your Reasonable Mind, as well as your Reasonable Mind thinking, actions, emotions, and sensations. What was your experience of your Reasonable Mind? In addition, describe the consequences or outcome of your Reasonable Mind taking control. Write about what would have been different had your Emotion Mind been in control.

Mindfulness "What" Skills Homework Sheet

Instructions: In the following spaces, describe your practice of each of these skills. For example, describe in detail your experience of Observe, Describe, and Participate. Practice Mindful Eating (i.e., practice using your Observe, Describe, and Participate skills while eating). Write about your Mindful Eating practice. Date each of your entries.

Observe

Describe

Participate

Mindfulness "How" Skills Homework Sheet

<u>Instructions:</u> In the following spaces, describe your practice of each of these skills. For example, describe observing Nonjudgmentally, and write about behaving One-Mindfully and Effectively. Use the "how" skills to practice Mindful Eating. Write about your Mindful Eating practice, including a date for each entry.

<u>Nonjudgmentally</u>

<u>One-Mindfully</u>

<u>Effectively</u>

Urge Surfing Homework Sheet

Urge Surfing involves mindful observing of urges to binge eat or to eat mindlessly. Urge Surfing involves stepping back from your experience and using Mindfulness skills, including nonjudgmental observing and describing of urges, cravings, and food preoccupation. Urge Surfing involves awareness without mindlessly giving in to the urge. Urge Surfing just notices without judging the urge, without pushing it away or holding onto it. One simply notices and describes, moment to moment, the ebb and flow of the urge without reacting to it.

Instructions: In the following space, describe your practice of Urge Surfing. Be very detailed. Describe your moment-to-moment observations. Describe the ebb and flow of your thoughts, feelings, sensations, urges.

Alternate Rebellion Homework Sheet

Alternate Rebellion is the opposite of cutting off your nose to spite your face. Alternate Rebellion involves the nonjudgmental observation of the desire or wish to rebel or retaliate. If your Wise Mind decision is to act on this desire, then Alternate Rebellion means doing it effectively without destroying your commitment to stop binge eating. Rebelling Effectively means not shooting yourself in the foot. You find an alternate means of rebellion that is effective and nondestructive. For example, you may decide to carry out your rebellion imaginally. Be creative in your rebellion. Act in a manner that maintains your self-respect.

Instructions: In the following space, write about your use of the Alternate Rebellion skill. Describe the circumstances surrounding the wish to rebel. Describe your thoughts, feelings, sensations, and behaviors. Describe in detail what you did to Effectively rebel. Describe how this was different from past rebellions in which you ended up harming yourself.

CHAPTER 5

Emotion Regulation Skills

At the heart of DBT for BED and BN is the underlying assumption that individuals who binge eat (and purge) frequently experience emotional states that they are ill equipped to skillfully manage. The aim of the Emotion Regulation skills taught in this module is to help clients acquire, develop, and implement adaptive skills that will enable them to more effectively manage negative emotional states, as well as cultivate a greater capacity for positive emotional experiences. Specifically, the Emotion Regulation skills (Appendix 5.1) and homework sheets outlined in this chapter are designed to enable the client to:

- Identify and label emotions.
- Understand the function of emotions.
- Reduce vulnerability to intense emotions.
- Increase the number of positive experiences.
- Increase mindfulness to emotions.
- Learn to change emotions when doing so would be effective.

It is important to emphasize that the goal of the Emotion Regulation skills is *not* to eliminate negative and unpleasant emotions. Distressing and difficult feelings are a part of life; they cannot be entirely avoided. However, clients often bring about or increase their distress and suffering through unskillful means. And this *can* be changed. The goal of the Emotion Regulation skills module is for clients to learn skillful emotion regulation strategies to reduce the suffering they create in their lives by, for example, turning to binge eating and other self-destructive behaviors. An equally important goal is to acquire and practice skills that build positive experiences and sense of self.

A second important point to underscore at the outset is the issue of judging emotions or binge-eating behaviors as either "good" or "bad." Judging in and of itself is not good or bad, right or wrong. One needs to use judgment in order to discern whether or not a particular behavior, action, or thought pattern will assist in achieving one's goals. Therefore, it is appropriate to question whether a particular action is skillful or unskillful for the purposes one has in mind. If one desires long-term happiness and well-being, being able to discern whether binge eating leads to this goal is useful. Additionally, if harsh or critical judging of one's emotions increases distress and decreases well-being, a goal would be to drop this type of judging. Ultimately, the question regarding judging is whether or not it is used skillfully in the service of one's goals.

DISCUSSION POINT:
"Any comments or reactions to these goals?"

MODEL FOR DESCRIBING EMOTIONS

An important first step in learning to effectively regulate emotions is developing the ability to identify and label all the various constituents of an emotional response. Doing so breaks down the emotional response into a series of components, facilitating a person's ability to understand what is happening and at which point he or she might effectively intervene. The model for describing emotions (Appendix 5.2) provides a schema for dissecting the various parts that make up the client's emotional response so that she or he will be better able to understand, change, control, modify, accept, or regulate her or his emotions.

Emotions are relatively short-lived phenomena. When an emotion lasts for a longer time, it is called a *mood*. An emotional response may be sustained if it becomes refired—for example, a client who is angry and ruminating may repeat the same inflammatory thoughts and images about the person with whom she or he is infuriated. Emotion Regulation skills are intended to help clients learn how to identify and interrupt unskillful sequences that contribute to unwanted emotion dysregulation.

Therapists use the model for describing emotions (Appendix 5.2) to highlight the complexity of emotions, which involve the interaction of multiple systems. When a client is anxious, for instance, the whole system is activated. The emotional experience includes changes in the brain, physical changes in the body, urges toward action, and so forth. Underscore for clients that the good news with regard to such a multifaceted system is that, by changing just one part of a response, clients can change their emotional experience. Because it may be more difficult to modify some components as opposed to others, the key—after identifying all the parts of the emotion—is to figure out which would be the easiest to change. That said, emphasize that this process is not effortless and requires perseverance and patience.

Therapists should reinforce the practice of Mindfulness skills in this context. For example, the Observe and Describe skills are important for identifying the trigger (prompting event) for an emotion. Emotions do not occur on their own; something always triggers an emotion. Identifying what prompted an emotion can be quite difficult, yet doing so is a critical skill to develop. Mindfulness skills such as Observe and Describe are key in this process.

Referring to the model, explain that prompting events may be internal triggers, including elements such as one's thoughts, memories, or physical sensations.

External events can also prompt an emotional response—for instance, if someone yells at the client or someone close to him or her dies. Prompting events can occur very rapidly and automatically, and therefore they can be challenging to detect. Like an iceberg, the greatest portion lies under the water and is difficult to see from the surface. Similarly, underneath the emotion that is palpable and visible, daily internal and external events that clients barely register may be those that actually trigger many of the emotions that lead to the client's binge eating (and purging). Clients will benefit by practicing becoming more aware of their prompting events lying "under the water."

Appendix 5.2 illustrates two ways in which prompting events may trigger emotions—directly or through an interpretation. Direct triggers, shown by the solid lines, are ones that automatically stimulate the client's entire emotion response system without his or her having to think about it. An example would be the experience of fear on seeing a gun pointed at one's face. Direct prompting events tend to be rare.

More typically, the prompting event involves an interpretation that triggers a client's emotional experience (as shown by the dashed line from Prompting Event 1 to Interpretation of Event). Explain that how one interprets or understands events will often depend on past learning and life experiences. For example, if you observed your mother reacting with fear whenever a dog appeared, you might develop the interpretation that dogs are always dangerous. Or, if you have experienced criticism for voicing your opinion, then you might interpret situations in which others ask for your opinion as highly risky and, therefore, feel anxious.

To further demonstrate the role of interpretations in emotional experiencing, suggest that clients imagine the following scenario: "You have made an arrangement to meet a friend. Upon seeing her, you notice she looks quite upset. Before inquiring what is wrong, how might you interpret your friend's apparent distress?" After eliciting responses, invite clients to consider how the various interpretations influenced their emotional experiences. Therapists may suggest that, in their experience, clients with eating disorders have a tendency to avoid conflict, but they may not always be accurate about identifying the actual occurrence of conflict. For example, a client might interpret the absence of a smiling face on a friend or spouse as an indication that the relationship is "in trouble," leading the client to feel depressed and/or anxious. Instead, the client's friend or spouse may simply be feeling cranky or annoyed for reasons having nothing to do with the client. The important point being emphasized is that how a client interprets events greatly influences her or his emotional response.

Once the prompting event and the consequent interpretation have occurred, a number of different reactions happen automatically and reflexively as part of the client's ongoing emotional experience. For example, brain changes, such as neurochemical signals, cause facial and body adjustments (e.g., alterations in body temperature, heart rate, muscle contraction), and an action urge (e.g., to run, hide) can be instantly triggered.

This discussion can help clients better understand the absurdity of instructing themselves to "stop feeling" an emotion. When nervous about an upcoming interview, for example, a client's interpretation of the event as threatening will automatically lead to physiological responses, including a rapid heart rate, a flushed feeling, and "gut clenching" nausea. Telling yourself not to experience these sensations would be like stepping into the rain without an umbrella and telling yourself to stop feeling the wetness on your head.

There are means by which clients can shut off awareness of their emotions—such as by using alcohol or food to produce sedative-like or activating effects. However, of course, the long-term cost of using these unskillful means is very high. Attempting to control one's emotional experience by binge eating to numb oneself or to shut off awareness of bodily cues and signals may backfire and result in emotions building in intensity (e.g., Gross, 2006). It is difficult to regulate emotions if one is avoiding or purposefully overlooking emotional cues and signals. Therefore, practice at registering bodily sensations of fatigue, anxiety, anger, and sadness early on in the emotional sequence may make these emotions easier to identify, understand, respond to, or manage.

◉ **DISCUSSION POINT:** *"Are you aware of your body's emotional signals or sensations? Please describe. Is binge eating and/or purging one of the ways you typically attempt to shut off awareness of your bodily cues? Which ones do you most typically attempt to ignore? Do they tend to be emotion-related sensations (e.g., anger, sadness), or are they more apt to be general body sensations, such as fatigue, hunger, or satiety?"*

One of the most important functions of emotions is communication using both nonverbal and verbal expressions. Individuals with eating disorders may likely attempt to regulate their emotions through attempts to stop or alter these expressive pathways. For example, a client might try to hide or conceal her or his facial expressions by smiling to cover or mask the fact that she or he is sad. Alternatively, a client might try to conceal her or his emotion by exaggerating her or his facial expressions. By taking on a somewhat theatrical or dramatic facial pattern, the client can actually conceal what she or he is truly feeling.

◉ **DISCUSSION POINT:** *"Is it difficult for others to receive messages about what you are feeling because you either restrict or exaggerate your emotional cues? Although there is nothing intrinsically good or bad about how you express your emotions, you might find it helpful to be aware of your tendencies so as to better consider the consequences."*

All the emotion components are included in the name given to the emotion (far right of Appendix 5.2). These components include those not observable to others that take place inside the client's body, such as brain chemistry, sensations, and urges, and those that are external and observable, such as body language, verbal language, and actions.

Naming an emotion facilitates emotion regulation. Acknowledging what one is experiencing is a first step toward control. Accurately naming an emotion validates one's emotional experience rather than allowing others to determine what one is experiencing or telling oneself what emotions "should" be present. This accurate naming can have an extremely powerful effect. Often, clients with eating disorders do not discriminate between their emotions. They tend to use automatic, global descriptors such as "I feel stressed" or "I feel bad." Therapists concede that taking the time to observe and describe one's emotions requires practice but that doing so will enable clients to figure out the precise feeling or feelings they are having, thus aiding them in regulating those feelings.

Emotions can have powerful aftereffects on a client's memory, thoughts, other emotions, and ability to function ("Aftereffects" box in Appendix 5.2). It is natural that an emotional response should not end with recognizing the emotion's name but instead stimulate additional thoughts, feelings, and reactions. The emotion's aftereffects can prompt the refiring of the same emotion or trigger a different emotional experience (Prompting Event 2 in Appendix 5.2). For example, the aftereffects of intense fear may temporarily paralyze a client's ability to think and act; an awareness of this immobility may trigger additional fear. Or the fear may prompt a different emotion, such as anger or shame. Therapists might say, "It is as if emotions are in love with themselves, particularly when they have established strong associations from past experiences." Emotions will frequently recur, firing and refiring, until a component in the response system changes. Clients need to intervene in only one aspect of the emotion response system in order to decrease, increase, or in some way change an entire emotional response. The key is to intervene skillfully so that the emotional response changes in the direction or manner one desires.

For individuals with eating disorders, a common aftereffect of an emotional response is to label the emotion as "stupid," instruct themselves to "snap out of it," or berate themselves by saying, "My feelings are wrong [or bad or shameful]." These self-critical and invalidating responses become a prompting event (Prompting Event 2 in Appendix 5.2) for increasing emotional intensity and often trigger a different emotion, such as shame, guilt, or depression. Research has found that judging one's emotions as invalid or wrong makes emotions even more intense (e.g., Gross, 2006). Blocking an emotion increases physiological arousal, which can lead to even greater urges to escape one's emotion by turning to food. Thus, although blocking or avoiding behaviors may distract one over the short run from feeling certain emotions, the long-term consequences are often a buildup of emotions and the generation of other, secondary emotions. These can have devastating consequences over time on the health, self-esteem, and general well-being of clients.

In order to be skillful in responding to one's emotions, it is important to distinguish between one's primary emotion (the original or first emotion felt) and one's secondary emotion (the emotion felt as a consequence of one's response to the primary emotion). Over 2,500 years ago, the Buddha recognized this phenomenon and stated that humans tend to cause themselves unnecessary suffering by shooting themselves with a second arrow. That is, the Buddha acknowledged that we cannot avoid all pain in life (getting shot with the first arrow) but that we *can* make wise choices and not cause ourselves additional pain by following the first arrow with a second! Unfortunately, all too often, individuals with eating disorders shoot that second arrow by responding to their own pain in negative, critical, and unskillful ways. Clients frequently fall into the trap of labeling their painful emotions rather than their responses to the emotions, such as binge eating and other maladaptive eating behaviors, as "the problem". Though painful emotions are often distressing, therapists point out that the problem is more correctly identified as attempting to block or numb the emotions. How one chooses to act or not act on his or her feelings is critical. It is possible to respond to primary painful feelings with understanding, interest, compassion, or myriad other skillful reactions that may lead to a decrease in emotion intensity and an increased sense of mastery.

DISCUSSION POINT: *"Think of a time when you had a primary emotion and a secondary emotion. Did your response to the primary emotion lead to feeling better . . . or cause more trouble and grief?"*

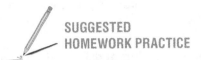

SUGGESTED
HOMEWORK PRACTICE

Therapists instruct clients to use the Primary Emotions and Secondary Reactions Homework Sheet (Appendix 5.3) to write about the experience of observing their primary and secondary emotions.

In order for clients to regulate their emotions effectively rather than turning to food, they must have a constructive relationship with their feelings. This will likely be a new experience. As clients probably recognize, individuals with eating disorders often use food to express their emotions. For example, they may express irritation with family members by sitting in front of the television with a bag of chips and a pint of ice cream and effectively walling themselves off.

Clients will also likely recognize that the type of relationship they have had with their feelings has been destructive to them and to their relationships with others. Therapists use this recognition to underscore the importance of practicing the skills of observing and describing the components that make up clients' emotional responses in order to help them build a more constructive relationship with their emotions. A useful guide for practicing observing and describing emotions is found in Linehan's (1993b, pp. 139–152) emotion regulation handout 4 on "Ways to Describe Emotions," a brief synopsis of which is given in Appendix 5.4.

In summary, the ability to identify emotions and their components can enhance the client's ability to regulate them. This involves identifying the prompting event for a client's emotion, her or his interpretation of the prompting event, her associated physical and body changes, emotional expression, and the aftereffects of the emotion. With increased awareness of these many components of her or his emotional response, the client has more opportunities to intervene and thus change her or his emotional response. For example, if a client notices muscle tension as part of her or his emotional response, she or he can stop and take a few deep breaths to relax. Or if a client notices that her or his interpretation of a situation is inflaming her or his emotional experience, she or he can practice considering alternative interpretations that would lessen the intensity of the emotion.

DISCUSSION POINT: *"Do you think that you use binge eating [and purging] as a way to express certain emotions, such as frustration or irritation? And/or does your binge eating serve to express certain action urges, such as the urge to rebel?"*

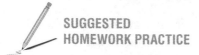

SUGGESTED
HOMEWORK PRACTICE

1. Therapists instruct clients to look over the Synopsis of Ways to Describe Emotions (Appendix 5.4), explaining that its purpose is to help clients confused about what they are feeling by giving examples of the components of universal emotions. Clients might begin by looking at the various emotion words to find the ones that best describe how they are feeling. They can then look over the prompting events to determine whether any apply and try to understand their relevance by using the examples of interpretations that often accompany that emotion. In this manner, clients may gain practice sorting through their emotional responses, including bodily expression, action urges, and so forth.

2. Therapists instruct clients to fill out the Observing and Describing Emotions Homework Sheet (Appendix 5.5, based on Linehan, 1993b, p. 162) about a recent emotional experience. (An example of a completed homework sheet is provided in Figure 5.1.) After having done so, clients should try to identify points at which they could have intervened to change their emotional experience. Therapists might suggest that clients select other colors of pen to write down other possible interpretations, other bodily experiences they might have had (e.g., relaxing the shoulders instead of tensing them), and other things they might have said or done. Clients should consider the emotions they might have experienced if, at the time, some of these emotional components had been altered. Might it have lessened the sense of intensity or urgency experienced or the untoward consequences?

TROUBLESHOOTING DIFFICULTIES
IN TEACHING THE MODEL OF EMOTIONS

• *Example*: "Can I have more than one emotion taking place at the same time?"

• *Potential therapist reply*: "Yes, you can. Sometimes you may experience more than one emotion in response to the same prompting event. At times these emotions can be in conflict with one another. Another possibility is that a secondary emotional reaction comes in quickly in response to the primary emotion, making things quite confusing and difficult to separate. If you experience two or more emotions, just practice observing and describing each."

MINDFULNESS OF YOUR CURRENT EMOTION

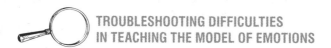

Therapists explain that applying core mindfulness skills in the service of accepting one's emotional experiences can reduce the suffering created from fighting, resisting, judging, and/or rejecting them (or ruminating, amplifying, and holding onto them). Because painful emotions are part of the human condition, everyone has to face negative feelings such as hatred, fear, anger, disappointment, betrayal, and jealousy—no matter how hard one might try not to. The trick is to find a way of relating to these painful and difficult feelings in a manner that does not increase suffering.

Observing and Describing Emotions Homework Sheet

EMOTION NAME(S) anger, frustration   **Intensity** (0–100) 100

PROMPTING EVENT for emotion (who, what, when, where):

Asked my husband to discuss how to pay for holiday gifts/trips this year. He refused to talk about it.

INTERPRETATIONS (beliefs, assumptions, appraisals) of situation:

(1) He wants me to not bother him and just handle it myself.

(2) He is trying to upset me.

[Alternative Interpretation—He's had a hard day at work & needed time to unwind. Not about me.]

BODY CHANGES and SENSING: What am I feeling in my body?

Felt tense, upset stomach, headache, hot.

BODY LANGUAGE: What is my facial expression? Posture? Gestures?

Sat rigidly in chair not facing him, frown on face.

ACTION URGES: What do I feel like doing? What do I want to say?

I wanted to scream or throw something to shake him up.

What **I SAID or DID** in the situation (Be specific):

I cried, tried to make him understand my worries for 30 min, then stomped out.

What **AFTEREFFECTS** does the emotion have on me (state of mind, other emotions, thoughts, etc.)?

Upset, flushed, frustrated, felt like there is no resolution, want to binge.

FUNCTION OF EMOTION:

(1) Self-validation of my position (2) Got me to try to communicate the situation (3) Gets me to try to find a solution

FIGURE 5.1. Example of a completed Observing and Describing Emotions Homework Sheet. Adapted from Linehan (1993b). Copyright 1993 by The Guilford Press. Adapted by permission.

Practicing the skill of Mindfulness of Your Current Emotion is a way clients can let go of emotional suffering. The Observe and Describe skills, as well as the skills of Nonjudgmentally and One-Mindfully, are very useful for helping to do this. The goal, as therapists describe, is to note the emotion's presence at the same time that the client steps back from it and gets "unstuck." Therapists remind clients that being mindful of the current emotion means being fully aware, open, and present oriented. One accepts the entirety of one's emotional experiences, rejecting none of it. One permits the feelings without trying to change or "fix" them. Mindfulness of Your Current Emotion does not mean that one *becomes* one's emotion—an important distinction. The therapist illustrates this by asking clients to imagine their emotion as a raging river. If one jumps into the river, one can be carried downstream by the rush of feeling. But if one remembers that it is possible to pause and sit on the bank, one has the option of observing and describing the emotion One-Mindfully and Nonjudgmentally. One can let the emotion rush by. In doing so, the client is not trying to suppress, block, or push the emotion away nor attempting to hold onto or amplify it.

Therapists might tell clients practicing this skill to specifically remind themselves that they are not their emotion. In other words, when experiencing very strong emotions, a client can remind him- or herself that this experience is not all of who he or she is but is an experience stemming from his or her current state of mind. Inevitably, all acute emotions pass. Therapists can illustrate this by asking clients to think about emotions that dominated their thoughts at one point but no longer do.

Mindfulness of Your Current Emotion is similar to the mindfulness skill of Urge Surfing (Chapter 4) in that the client is riding an emotion's wave and staying with the emotional experience as it rises, crests, and falls—without fighting the wave or trying to stop it. Use the following script (modifying as needed) to lead clients in the related experiential exercise.

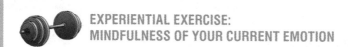

EXPERIENTIAL EXERCISE:
MINDFULNESS OF YOUR CURRENT EMOTION

"Take a moment to sit in your chair, feet on the floor, posture erect, breathing slow, easy breaths from your diaphragm. Find a place for your eyes to focus, or let them gently close. Then bring to mind a strong emotion that you have been aware of recently. Maybe you were really hurt or angry? Or very sad? Whatever this strong emotion, try to imagine letting go of the suffering by observing your emotion. Imagine stepping back from it, getting unstuck, and watching it. Experience the emotion as a wave, letting it come and go just as waves crash to the shore on the beach and then are pulled away. Do not try and block the wave. Do not try to amplify it. Fully accept whatever is present without adding to it. Practice releasing or unhanding the experience. Then take several deep flowing breaths and end the exercise."

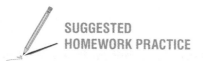

SUGGESTED
HOMEWORK PRACTICE

Therapists instruct clients to practice being mindful of their current emotion by using the Mindfulness "What" skills of Observe and Describe and the "How" skills of Nonjudgmentally and One-Mindfully.

Loving Your Emotions

Therapists introduce this new skill by reminding clients that the Mindfulness skills leave the door open for all of the client's experiences. They allow awareness without judgment or condemnation. With acceptance, the client is allowed a "pure" experience. He or she may have pain but does not add to it the extra baggage that results when he or she fights or resists the emotion. Although it is absolutely natural to want as little pain as possible, according to the research-supported view described, attempts to suppress or avoid pain simply add to the suffering and distress one experiences.

Therapists may find it helpful to illustrate this concept by having clients recall the Chinese straw "finger puzzle" (*en.wikipedia.org/wiki/Chinese_finger_trap*). The puzzle teaches that fighting to get your fingers out from both ends of a straw cylinder ensures that you stay locked in a struggle, whereas letting go and ceasing to pull on your fingers releases you from the puzzle trap. Therapists might also describe a monkey trap that uses no restraints or clamps. The trap contains a hole through which the monkey can reach a banana. The hole is just large enough for a monkey's arm, but not for both a monkey's arm *and* a banana. By being unwilling to release its grip on the banana, the monkey is not able to free its arm and thus is trapped. But as soon as a monkey accepts the reality of the situation and its limits by releasing the banana, the monkey is no longer stuck.

The story of the ugly duckling, with its message of accepting who one is rather than trying to be someone else, is also relevant. Just like the ugly duckling that turned out to be a swan, all of a client's emotions are part of her or his experience. Some might seem ugly to the client, others beautiful. But there can be some meaning and wisdom even in those emotions that seem like "ugly ducklings." Similarly, the skill of acceptance allows clients to observe and describe their emotion, radically accepting its presence instead of using food to try to avoid experiencing it.

Therapists will find it helpful to acknowledge that radically accepting, let alone loving, one's emotions is likely one of the hardest skills for clients with eating disorders to practice. The word "loving" often raises judgments that therapists should encourage clients to vocalize. Initially, clients may find it easier to practice radical acceptance of their emotions. This acceptance is not a superficial one but a very deep, internal, Wise Mind acceptance of one's emotion.

It is important to convey understanding of how hard it is for many clients to let go of trying to control their feelings, emphasizing that this skill requires a great deal of practice. Also make clear that clients who do learn should find themselves able to focus their energy more productively. Therapists might offer the metaphor of having a leak in the oil pan of your car. One option in that situation is to spend all your energy thinking about how much you are suffering by having to continually check the oil level and purchase new oil. Therapists ask whether clients are able to recognize that staying engaged in the struggle is actually a distraction from thinking about the larger issues of why one has the oil leak in the first place or how to go about fixing it. Thinking about the cause of the problem or how to solve it is also not pleasant, but it is likely to be a much more effective strategy.

Following is a script for an experiential exercise illustrating this skill that we have used in our groups (to be modified as needed).

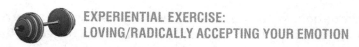

EXPERIENTIAL EXERCISE:
LOVING/RADICALLY ACCEPTING YOUR EMOTION

"Begin by sitting comfortably in your chair, letting it fully support you. Keep your spine straight, head up, and find a place for your eyes to focus. Take a few deep flowing breaths, in and out. Then practice radical acceptance of who you are and of your emotional experience. Practice not judging but allowing yourself to accept whatever is there, even if it is painful and you wish you did not feel it. Let it be just what it is. Do this while breathing in and out for ten breaths. Then end the exercise."

DISCUSSION POINT: *"What do you think about radically accepting your emotions, being willing to be open to all of your feelings? Which emotions are you not accepting? Can you think of a time when radical acceptance of your emotion has reduced your level of suffering?"*

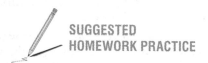

SUGGESTED
HOMEWORK PRACTICE

Therapists instruct clients to practice letting go of emotional suffering by radically accepting their emotions. Clients should track their practice of this skill on their diary cards.

FUNCTION OF EMOTIONS

Introduce this section by explaining that evidence pointing to the important function that emotions serve is their presence beginning at birth. Crying, frowning, trembling, and laughing are hardwired, so to speak, into our nervous systems. One cannot just get rid of them.

Acknowledge that because emotions are functional to the individual, changing binge eating (and purging) behaviors can be very difficult, especially when such behaviors serve important communication purposes and/or provide a sense of temporary relief. It is therefore especially important for a client to understand how her or his emotions function, as this knowledge can help her or him be more effective at changing the emotion or her or his responses to it. This is a key reason clients will be learning about the function of their emotions in this session.

Therapists explain that emotions and emotional behavior generally serve the following purposes: (1) to communicate to others and influence their behavior, (2) to organize and motivate the client's own behavior, and (3) to validate the client's own perceptions and interpretation of events. Each is discussed in turn.

Emotions Communicate and Influence Others

Therapists describe how the expressive characteristics of emotion in the client's voice, face, gestures, posture, and words serve the essential function of communicating his or her emotional state to others. The value in these communications is both that it allows others to know how he or she feels and that it influences the behavior of others. The facial expressions and gestures linked with one's emotions communicate information very rapidly. Compared with words, emotions can be faster, more powerful, and more effective at influencing others, such as when a person's terrified face signals a panic or a baby's sharp cry calls forth the attention and nurturance of its caregiver.

When nonverbal expressions, such as posture and facial expressions, do not match what a person states verbally, others usually will trust the person's nonverbal expressions over his or her verbal ones. This "mismatched" communication can be very confusing, however, for both the sender and the receiver of the communication. For example, if a client verbally insists, "No, I'm fine, nothing is bothering me" when her or his facial muscles are tense and body slumped, others may be aware that something is wrong but may interpret the client's verbal message as indicating that she or he wishes to be left alone. This may lead them to change the subject and collude with the client's statement that nothing is wrong—potentially leading the client's emotional experience to a greater intensity (e.g., feeling more hurt and uncared for).

The therapist points out that because communication is an essential function of emotions, it can be very hard for clients to change an emotional experience until the communication has been accomplished. Thus one means of changing an emotion is to communicate with a person who is receptive, allowing time for the intensity of the emotion to diminish.

Therapists will find it useful to point out to clients that whether or not it is intentional, their emotions will influence others. The more aware a client is of what she or he is feeling, the more direct her or his communication can be.

Emotions Organize and Motivate for Action

Another chief function of emotion is to organize and motivate the client's behavior—to get her or him to run, hide, cling, fight, and so forth. This function has survival value and is an important reason that therapists are not suggesting that clients attempt to rid themselves of all emotion! Fear, for example, may keep clients from engaging in acts that are dangerous. The threat of shame may keep clients from behaving in ways that could risk their losing the attachment of significant others.

Emotions have the capacity to activate certain behaviors within us in which we otherwise might not engage. For example, fear can cause the brave to cower, or anger may drive the pacifist to fight. Joy → action/liberation

⊙ **DISCUSSION POINT:** *"Can you think of any current examples of emotions (e.g., anger, excitement, shame, guilt, fear) that may be functioning to organize you, prepare you, and/ or motivate your actions?"*

Therapists consider with clients how binge eating (and purging) interferes with the organizing, preparing, and motivating function of their emotions. For example, a client might imagine having an argument with a friend or spouse, after which she or he felt sad and experienced regret. Such emotions might motivate the client to communicate an apology or to find some means of repairing the rift. If, instead, the client turns to food to suppress her or his sadness and guilt and subsequently withdraws, the function of communicating an apology is interfered with, and the client may ultimately feel even worse.

 DISCUSSION POINT: *"In what way do you think binge eating and/or purging interferes with your ability to effectively manage your emotions?"*

Emotions Communicate to Ourselves

Therapists describe another function of emotions: to communicate information to ourselves. A client's emotional reactions, including his or her "gut" response or intuition about a situation, can give him or her invaluable knowledge. Emotions can act as signals and sometimes even alarms.

Although emotions can usefully support a client's reactions, clients must also be made aware of the possible inaccurate influence of emotions as an information source. In other words, the client might depend solely on her or his Emotion Mind reasoning when assessing or reacting to a situation instead of taking into account her or his Reasonable Mind reasoning. One explanation for this tendency involves the ongoing influence of the past on the present, as brought up earlier. A client whose parent was afraid of spiders, for example, might grow up thinking all spiders are dangerous—even though most are harmless. In such a case, if the client reacts with panic when she or he sees a spider, this panic communicates to her or him the potential of danger but would not necessarily be accurate for the situation. In other words, the client is using her or his emotions to confirm what her or his Emotion Mind is telling her or him, instead of searching for a fuller Wise Mind understanding.

Many instinctive anxiety and fear reactions stem from this ongoing emotional influence of the past on the present. For example, if someone does not say hello to a person when passing him or her on the street, it would not necessarily be a cause for alarm in and of itself. But if the person has a history of being ignored by his or her parents, he or she might interpret a current situation as a signal of being unlovable. His or her emotions can still serve a useful function as long as the person recognizes that in such cases his or her emotions are communicating about the past rather than the present. Indeed, recognizing the way in which our emotions communicate information regarding how we feel about the past can help us understand why certain intense emotions can be triggered by seemingly trivial prompting events.

 DISCUSSION POINT: *"Take a moment to think about times when your emotions are giving you information about a situation versus giving you information based on your past learning experiences."*

Although there are helpful ways that emotions communicate to us, therapists draw clients' attention to additional examples of how overreliance on one's emotions can lead to difficulties. When a client uses her or his emotional reactions to *confirm* what she or he already believes to be true, it is difficult for her or him to appraise situations objectively. Examples include: "Because I feel worthless, then I *must* actually be worthless"; "If I am furious with my boss, then he *must* be an insensitive tyrant"; or "If I feel angry with you, it proves you *must* be wrong."

Understandably in such instances, as therapists explain, modifying one's intense negative emotions can feel especially invalidating. This presents a difficult situation for clients. The way out of the trap is for clients to validate their entitlement to feel exactly as they do (e.g., legitimizing their "right" to feel angry) while simultaneously accepting the facts or the reality of the situation (e.g., that aspects of the other person's argument may be accurate).

⊙ **DISCUSSION POINT:** *"Have there been times when you treated as facts the information provided by your emotions? Would changing the negative emotions have felt invalidating? Can you recognize any links to binge eating?"*

Therapists may find it helpful to emphasize the following, particularly for clients having difficulty validating their emotions. Having emotions is part of what it means to be a human being. As noted, one's emotions are biologically hardwired responses. At the most basic level, emotions must be acknowledged in the same way one acknowledges sensations such as heat from the sun or moisture from the rain. As brought up earlier, trying to ignore the existence of uncomfortable emotions would be like saying, "I don't like the sensation of feeling wet, so I'm going to pretend my hair isn't soaked with water." Unless one is willing to acknowledge an emotion, he or she cannot decide what to do. Ignoring the fact that one's head is wet, for example, means that one cannot assess the situation objectively before reacting (e.g., determining whether the water is due to a leaky roof or a fire sprinkler going off due to a fire).

Therapists underscore that the client's *wish* to rid her- or himself of discomfort is always valid. Wanting to bypass experiencing a distressing emotion and its related urges through binge eating is an understandable desire. But now the client has other options for comforting her- or himself that hold promise of being ultimately more effective. Learning to think about the function of the emotion rather than just trying to get rid of it or diminish awareness of it is an effective strategy in itself.

JUSTIFIED VERSUS UNJUSTIFIED EMOTIONS

Therapists convey their belief in the usefulness of a concept that may be new to the client—that of justified versus unjustified emotions. This concept does not invalidate the earlier discussion that all emotions are valid; but whether an emotion is *justified* depends on whether it is warranted by the particulars of a situation. Therapists explain that, for example, feeling panic during a severe earthquake would be considered a justified emotion. It may not be *effective* for a client, who may still wish to regulate her or his experience of that emotion so as to be able to think and act as clearly as possible, but the emotion *itself* is justified. On the other hand, feeling that same amount of panic on entering an elevator is *unjustified* because the actual likelihood of danger is very, very low. Again, this is *not* the same as saying the emotion is invalid or wrong. The emotion may be highly understandable, perhaps being based on having once been trapped in an elevator. But it is considered unjustified based on its timing (i.e., if the current situation does not warrant it) or on its intensity not being appropriate to the circumstances.

Therapists describe how the ability to distinguish between justified and unjustified emotions can enable the client to step back from being caught up in her or his emotions. Validating her or his emotion while simultaneously recognizing the effectiveness of regulating its intensity is a highly useful skill. Therapists caution, however, that it is not useful for a client to become overly caught up in distinguishing between justified and unjustified emotions, as there can be instances in either case in which it makes sense for the client to try to change his or her emotion. For example, rescue team members working during the unstable conditions of an earthquake may feel fear, which is justified given the situation, yet may wish to reduce its intensity in order to more effectively perform their jobs.

Binge Eating (and Purging) as an Emotional Expression

Therapists may wish to take this moment to step back and review with clients the assumption, fundamental to this treatment approach, that a client's binge eating and other problem eating behaviors are components of her or his emotional response system. Specifically, like the action of fleeing when afraid, binge eating can be understood as part of the "action component" of an emotional response. The client's binge eating (and purging) may serve many purposes, including communicating to others, influencing others, and communicating to oneself—whether the client intends these things or not. Because of the way binge eating functions for the client, changing her or his behavior, despite her or his strong desire to do so, can feel extremely challenging, and the client should not lose heart. Therapists explain that binge eating (and purging) has been a "quick fix" or short-term means of regulating her or his emotions. But as the client is well aware, the effects of this type of "fix" dissipate quickly. Practicing and applying the Emotion Regulation skills in treatment requires more time, but therapists emphasize that its benefits may last, without the many debilitating negative consequences of binge eating.

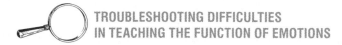 **TROUBLESHOOTING DIFFICULTIES IN TEACHING THE FUNCTION OF EMOTIONS**

- *Example 1*: "Why would I want to hold onto an emotion if it distorts my perspective?"

- *Potential therapist reply*: "People often hold onto their emotions because they are afraid that if they let them go, they won't have had a right to feel the way that they do; they will have been 'wrong.' Recognizing the function of one's emotion can be very helpful when you realize there *are* reasons for the way you feel, whether or not the reasons are apparent, and these reasons exist even when you decide it is in your best interest to change how you feel. For example, imagine someone is criticizing you and you are angry. You don't want to feel this level of fury, but you don't know how to let go of your anger without also losing your justification for having it. The trick is to find a way to validate your emotions while maintaining perspective regarding the reality of your situation. This involves learning to hold onto the dialectic between many opposing truths that are simultaneously possible. For example, it's possible to believe you are right but not to hold onto your intense anger, just as it's possible to feel some anger while also acknowledging that potentially the other person has a point. The goal of this treatment is to help you understand the function of emotions so that you don't turn to binge eating as a way to 'solve' a conflict through numbing your feelings or by using a secondary emotion, such as becoming angry or ashamed at yourself, to block your primary emotion."

• *Example 2*: "Are you saying that we should always reduce our intense emotions?"

• *Potential therapist reply*: "We are only referring to situations in which it would be effective to change or to reduce your emotion's intensity rather than engaging in binge eating and/or purging as a way of numbing. We aren't suggesting you should always want to reduce the intensity of your emotions."

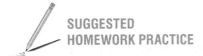

SUGGESTED HOMEWORK PRACTICE

Encourage clients by reminding them that identifying the function of their emotions, as well as continuing to practice observing and describing these emotions, can significantly help to reduce their binge eating (and purging) and other problematic eating-related behaviors.

1. Therapists instruct clients to fill out an "emotion diary" to gain experience in thinking about the function of emotions. Clients should list five emotion entries per week and, for each, identify one or more of the emotion's functions. Clients may choose the strongest emotion felt on a particular day or perhaps one experienced as particularly troubling.

2. Therapists instruct clients to complete the Observing and Describing Emotions Homework Sheet (Appendix 5.5) for at least three of the five emotion diary entries.

3. Therapists ask clients to observe what happens after they attempt to identify the function of their distressing emotions. Communicating about the emotion to oneself, for instance, sometimes helps to reduce its intensity. If the client does not notice this effect, he or she might consider communicating the emotion to someone else or allowing the function of the emotion to be expressed via a more effective means than binge eating (and purging).

REDUCING VULNERABILITY TO EMOTION MIND

The rationale for teaching the skills in this section is that binge eating, purging, and other problematic eating behaviors are more likely to be used when the client is in Emotion Mind and her or his emotions are dysregulated. Hence, identifying and changing factors that make a client more vulnerable to her or his Emotion Mind is key.

Check with clients about patterns they may have noticed regarding their vulnerability to engage in binge eating. Typically, clients realize that during times when they are tired, ill, and/or extremely hungry, they are more emotionally reactive and more likely to turn to food to soothe themselves. By targeting the specific behaviors that make them more vulnerable to Emotion Mind, clients can begin to break the links between those behaviors and problematic eating.

Six guidelines for reducing emotional vulnerability are discussed in this section (and described in greater detail in Emotion Regulation Handout 6 in Linehan, 1993b, p. 154). While reviewing these guidelines, therapists help clients to identify their emotional vulnerabilities, to observe and describe how these influence their emotional reactivity, and to increase their awareness of how these factors intensify their problem eating behaviors. Suggested probes are offered here. Having identified the specific areas of vulnerability, therapists encourage clients to think through ways to address these vulnerability factors in the future.

Treating Physical Illness

"Do you notice patterns of turning to food when feeling physically unwell?" Many clients with eating disorders have a tendency, as mentioned, to distract themselves from awareness of their bodies. "Do you try to ignore your body's messages when feeling sick so as to be able to function the same as always?" Ask clients to think through the costs of such behaviors. "Can you afford to keep paying this price? Compared with treating physical illness directly, how does binge eating [and purging] affect your short- and long-term functioning? What behaviors need to change in order to reduce this source of vulnerability?"

Balancing Eating

"Do you notice a link between your emotions and not eating properly—eating too much, too little, or eating food with too little nutritive content ('junk' food)?" For many clients, eating poorly can lead to feeling more grouchy and irritable. Balanced eating requires awareness of the link between how one eats and one's vulnerability to negative emotions. "What patterns do you notice, whether in the short or long run, that are associated with your having greater emotional vulnerability?"

Avoiding Mood-Altering Drugs

Therapists review with clients how certain substances (e.g., caffeine, alcohol) may influence a client's mood. For instance, does caffeine cause the client's body to be more agitated, less calm? What is alcohol's effect on their bodies? Is the client more likely to binge (and purge), for example, after drinking alcohol? Does the client use any other mood-altering drugs, and, if so, what is their relationship to the client's vulnerability to binge eating (and purging) and other problematic food behaviors?

Balancing Sleep

Therapists emphasize that sleep is essential for the client's emotional stability. When one is tired, one becomes more emotionally vulnerable and, therefore, more susceptible to bingeing (and purging). Often clients will admit to using food to increase their energy levels. "Do you try to mask fatigue with food rather than responding to fatigue directly by taking a nap or getting more sleep? Is this working for you? If not, what changes might you be willing to make?"

Getting Exercise

For clients with a tendency to eat when feeling depressed, lack of exercise can be a particular source of vulnerability. Increasing activity and physical stamina can be an effective route to improving one's mood, reducing stress levels, and increasing one's sense of well-being. Therapists remind clients that changing one's behavior can change one's emotional experience. When depressed or discouraged, becoming more active can help to shift one's state of mind toward being less despondent. Therapists explain that exercise is a mood-independent behavior in that it is not tightly linked to one's emotions. Indeed, exercise can act to change one's mood and reduce emotional vulnerability. Therapists convey clearly that getting moderate exercise does not require running a marathon nor pushing oneself to the point of injury. It means, in a balanced way, doing something to get one's limbs moving, such as a walk, swim, or bike ride. "Do you have a regular exercise program? What has been your experience with exercise? Does exercise affect your mood, binge-eating patterns, and/or purging behaviors?"

Building Mastery

Therapists describe building mastery as performing activities that increase confidence and lead to a sense of competence. Feeling more satisfied and fulfilled decreases the client's vulnerability to negative emotions such as depression. Therapists may need to work with the client to identify activities that require some degree of effort, are somewhat challenging, and help the client to build self-esteem and satisfaction. Therapists underscore that engaging in such activities each day is key, because actually doing these confidence-enhancing endeavors (not just thinking about them) gives new and different feedback to the client's brain, thereby helping to change her or his emotional experience. Like exercise, building mastery is a mood-independent behavior. It might involve doing something creative, such as making jewelry. Especially for binge-eating clients who are overweight, exercising is an excellent activity that helps to build mastery. "Can you think of activities that would build mastery for you?"

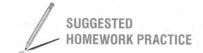

1. Therapists instruct clients to review the six domains for reducing their vulnerability to Emotion Mind. Clients should make specific plans to reduce their vulnerability within each pertinent domain. For example, if too little sleep is a problem, clients might make it a goal to get at least 8 hours' sleep for 5 of the next 7 days.

2. Clients should fill out their goals in the Reduced Vulnerability to Emotion Mind section of the Steps for Reducing Painful Emotions Homework Sheet (Appendix 5.6, adapted from the Emotion Regulation Homework Sheet 3 in Linehan, 1993b, p. 164). (An example of a completed homework sheet is provided in Figure 5.2.)

STEPS FOR INCREASING POSITIVE EMOTIONS

Therapists introduce the basic assumption that usually there are good reasons to explain why individuals experience negative emotions such as unhappiness and depression. One is that an imbalance exists between the number of negative experiences clients have in their lives compared with the number of positive experiences. Another common reason is that clients do not focus attention on and fully experience the positive emotions they do have. Both of these are discussed in greater detail in this section.

Increasing Daily Pleasant Experiences

Therapists check with clients regarding whether the assumption holds true for them and, if so, whether this skewed ratio creates unhappiness. Perhaps clients have even learned to expect negative experiences. If therapists obtain agreement, they state explicitly that clients who wish to experience more happiness will have to put considerable effort into creating more positive experiences. No one is very happy when not engaging in activities that are positive, meaningful, fulfilling, and satisfying. Like saving pennies in a piggy bank, clients will have to accumulate or invest in many positive experiences to reap rewards.

Emphasize the key role of balance when clients begin to think about creating more happiness for themselves. Just as clients cannot work all day every single day, they cannot lie out and relax on a beautiful beach all day every single day. As therapists explain, experience with clients with eating disorders leads them to assume that a client's imbalance is usually one of having too few pleasant events, which can then increase the likelihood of their turning to food as a way of coping with overwhelming negative emotions.

Explain that the idea behind the Adult Pleasant Events Schedule (see Appendix 5.7 for an abbreviated version of Linehan's [1993b, pp. 157–159] Emotion Regulation Handout 8) is that there are myriad activities clients could engage in daily to increase positive events and potentially positive feelings. Clients may not be engaging in enough of these to outweigh the negative or neutral events in their lives.

For each Emotion Regulation skill, check whether you used it during the week and describe what you did. Write on back of page if you need more room.

REDUCED VULNERABILITY TO EMOTION MIND: Treated physical illness? ✓
                                                  Balanced eating? ✓
                                                  Avoided mood-altering drugs?
                                                  Balanced sleep? ✓
                                                  Exercised? ✓
                                                    Practiced mastery?

I had a bad cold and took care of myself. Went to bed on time each night (and extra early when ill). Walked with my friend two evenings this past week for exercise. Focused on eating healthy meals with reasonable portions each day.

INCREASED POSITIVE EVENTS
Increased daily pleasant activities (circle):   M (T) W   TH (F) S (SUN)   (Describe)
Listened to music during eve (Tues), took bubble bath (Fri), took pottery class (Sun).

LONG-TERM GOALS worked on:
Goal is to start dating again—(1) Took a picture for online profile, (2) worked on profile, (3) asked friends for recommendations of good dating activities.

ATTENDED TO RELATIONSHIPS:
Called good friend from high school for first time in months to catch up. Told sister I loved her and wanted to work on improving our relationship.

AVOIDED AVOIDING (Describe)
Went to bank and got my account balance. Got on scale.

MINDFULNESS OF POSITIVE EXPERIENCES THAT OCCURRED
  ✓   Focused (and refocused) attention on positive experiences?
  ✓   Distracted from worries about positive experience?

MINDFULNESS OF THE CURRENT EMOTION
  ✓   Observed the emotion?   ✓   Remembered:
  ✓   Experienced the emotion?   Not to act on emotion?
                                                          Times I've felt different?

OPPOSITE ACTION: How did I act opposite to the current emotion?
I've been feeling sad and ashamed about how much I weigh. Had urge to binge and sit at home. Instead, I got out and went shopping for clothes I feel more attractive in.

FIGURE 5.2. Example of a Steps for Reducing Painful Emotions Completed Homework Sheet. Adapted from Linehan (1993b). Copyright 1993 by The Guilford Press. Adapted by permission.

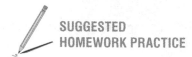

SUGGESTED
HOMEWORK PRACTICE

Therapists instruct clients to choose at least one positive event each day over the following week in which to participate. Clients should keep track of such events, perhaps using a homework sheet such as Appendix 5.6.

Building Long-Term Positive Events

Consider with clients how binge eating and other problem eating behaviors interfere with their ability to engage in and enjoy pleasant events in both the short and long term and how having more pleasant events might help decrease their turning to eating. Request that clients identify long-term goals they believe would contribute to their experiencing more satisfying, fulfilling lives that would bring them more happiness than they have currently. What small steps does each client need to make to reach these goals?

Attending to Relationships

Talk over with clients the assumption that most individuals need good relationships to be happy and to have meaningful lives. What do clients need to do to attend to the relationships in their lives? What could they do to make their relationships more rewarding? How does binge eating (and purging) interfere with these relationships?

Avoid Avoiding

Point out how no one feels very positive if she or he is avoiding problem solving or avoiding doing necessary things. Feeling masterful requires an active and positive engagement with one's life. As therapists explain, "Avoiding is similar to capitulating, convincing yourself that there is absolutely no other choice than to use food in a given situation." Passive avoidance or capitulating, as opposed to increasing feelings of mastery, usually leads to negative feelings. The skill of Avoid Avoiding involves actively blocking the option to misuse food (or engage in other problematic behaviors) as an avoidance strategy.

Increasing Mindfulness of Positive Experiences

Clients with eating disorders, besides making too little time for positive events, tend also to be highly skilled at destroying the positive emotions they *do* have with worry, guilt, self-punishment, and self-condemnation. Doing so has the effect of wiping out these positive experiences, leaving clients with only fleeting moments of positive feelings. Therapists discuss, therefore, the reason that one of the skills being taught is to be Mindful of Positive Experiences, letting them endure, instead of spoiling your fun (so to speak) with secondary emotional reactions.

Clients, for example, may be laughing and enjoying themselves, only to destroy that pleasure with a sense of shame that "I'm being too loud." In other words, clients with problematic eating behaviors will typically undercut their sense of pride and accomplishment with feelings of guilt (e.g., "I should not feel happy if others are not happy" or "I should not experience pride about my own accomplishments if someone else has been unsuccessful").

DISCUSSION POINT: *"Are you someone who makes time for pleasant events but limits the potential to derive enjoyment from your activities by engaging in self-criticism, guilt, and worry?"*

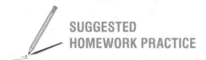

SUGGESTED HOMEWORK PRACTICE

1. Therapists instruct clients to consider positive feelings they would like to increase (e.g., pride, joy, love) and to identify ways in which their secondary reactions may be interfering with deriving full enjoyment.

2. Therapists instruct clients to practice attending to positive experiences and refocusing their attention when worries or other secondary emotions intrude. Therapists might say, "All emotions come and go, including positive emotional experiences. The idea is to not destroy or distract oneself from the positive emotions before they have had a chance to fully exist."

3. Therapists instruct clients to set up specific goals for the different guidelines intended to increase positive emotions (e.g., attending to relationships, avoid avoiding, building mastery). Using a homework sheet (e.g., Appendix 5.6), clients should write down a specific first small step (or series of small steps) they could take during the following week to work on achieving these goals. Their progress should be tracked.

The following suggested questions may be asked to check on homework related to reducing emotional vulnerability:

- "Did making specific behavioral changes help reduce your vulnerability to emotion mind and to problem eating?"
- "What was the effect of increasing positive events, both in the short run and longer term? How did practicing mindfulness of your positive experiences influence your sense of emotional vulnerability?"
- "What would you identify as your strengths and weaknesses in these areas? How can you reduce your areas of weakness by positive endeavors?"

ACTING OPPOSITE TO THE CURRENT EMOTION

The goal of learning this skill is to be able to change or regulate one's emotions by acting in a way that is opposite to one's current emotion. Acquisition of this skill offers clients a very powerful means of changing their emotions over the long term.

Therapists make clear that the very first question to address when practicing this skill is whether a person wants to change his or her emotion. The skill of acting opposite to an emotion is not intended to be used when an emotion is adaptive and justified. Rather, it is for instances in which an emotion is ineffective and getting in the way of experiencing one's desired quality of life. As was described earlier, certain emotions may not be justified in the sense that they do not fit the facts of one's situation. A client's fear of air travel, for example, may be out of proportion to the actual danger of flying and may interfere with important life goals, such as keeping in touch with family and friends in other parts of the country or the world. Or an emotion is justified but its presence or intensity may be ineffective or maladaptive for one's circumstances. At such times, it may be effective for clients to change their emotions.

Therapists review with clients that there are many skillful ways to change an emotional experience, including considering alternative interpretations, thinking about the function of one's emotion, and so forth. Acting Opposite to a Current Emotion is a behaviorally based skill for changing one's emotional experience. Acting Opposite is not the same as "masking" one's emotion or covering it over. One can validate one's emotions while making a Wise Mind decision to act opposite to them.

A next step is for clients to identify the natural action behavior associated with the emotion they wish to change. The action to take is then to behave opposite to that natural action urge. The natural action behavior associated with the emotion of fear, for example, is to attempt to escape or avoid. To change the emotion of fear, clients must do the opposite of running away; they must *approach*. To overcome the fear of airplane travel, for example, clients must fly on planes—*over* and *over* and *over*.

Therapists highlight two important tips for applying the skill of Acting Opposite to the Current Emotion. First of all, as cannot be overemphasized, clients should use this skill only for emotions that are interfering with their desired quality of life (i.e., are not effective). The client would not employ Acting Opposite when encountering a justified fear that is adaptive for a dangerous situation.

Second, clients must remember that Acting Opposite to the Current Emotion will not provide an immediate emotional change. Indeed, the intensity of one's emotion will, in the short term, increase. For example, if clients are phobic about spiders and begin acting opposite and approaching arachnids, the emotions of anxiety and fear will spike at first. The fastest way to reduce fear and anxiety is by avoiding spiders. But, as therapists caution, avoidance acts to strengthen the fear response because essentially one is telling oneself that one's interpretation of danger when encountering spiders is correct. Avoidance makes it more likely in subsequent situations that one will experience fear. Research in this area has demonstrated that, in the long term, acting opposite to emotions of fear, depression, and anxiety is an effective strategy. The emotions *do* change.

Underscore that practicing Acting Opposite to the Current Emotion is not a quick-fix skill that yields results immediately or that will work despite being practiced only once or even a few times. Particularly when trying to change very intense or well-established emotions, repetition is key. Beginning with the first time clients act opposite, their brain begins processing new information. On that level, change is taking place right away, but time is required to enable that initial brain processing to change the emotion the client experiences. It is vital for clients to be prepared so as not to be unrealistic and risk becoming too easily discouraged.

Furthermore, important in the success of Acting Opposite is not only repetition but also full participation in Acting Opposite (Acting Opposite *all the way*). This requires both physically engaging in the action that is opposite to the urge and also altering one's thoughts (e.g., judgments). In other words, practicing opposite action also involves Acting Opposite with thoughts and nonverbal behaviors.

Review with clients what Acting Opposite entails for each of the basic emotions.

Fear

Acting Opposite to fear means approaching the feared situation over and over and over. When fear is overwhelmingly intense, clients should attempt to divide the feared tasks into a series of smaller steps. Then clients would approach the first step on the list, then the second, and so forth. For example, a client with a fear of air travel might break down Acting Opposite by first going to an airport to sit and watch the planes take off and arrive. The therapist emphasizes that approaching, small step by small step, what feels overwhelming will ultimately give clients a sense of control and mastery.

Therapists might ask clients to think about things that make them anxious (e.g., asking for help, accepting help when offered) and take steps to approach rather than give in to those fears.

Guilt and Shame

It is important to help clients distinguish between justified versus unjustified guilt and shame, as these are treated differently. Explain that guilt and shame are justified when a client's actions violate her or his core Wise Mind values. If clients engage in cheating and if guilt and shame fit their Wise Mind values, repair is the solution to changing the emotion. Clients will likely need to consult their Wise Mind to gain clarity about what this repair involves. To change the emotion of justified guilt and shame, therefore, clients must acknowledge that their behavior violated their values and must repair the damage, accept the consequences, and finally forgive themselves and move on.

Therapists emphasize that *accepting the consequences of one's action does not mean judging oneself as bad*. It is an unavoidable fact of life that everyone makes mistakes and does things they wish they had not done. Clients often become "stuck" in guilt and shame because they are afraid that admitting to wrongdoing and repairing the transgression would mean having to hate themselves. Accepting consequences can be very freeing if it can be done without judgment.

When clients' behaviors do not violate their core Wise Mind values, the emotions of guilt and shame are probably unjustified. Likely, these emotions are based on fear. For example, clients who experience guilt and shame when saying no to a request are likely reacting to the emotion of fear—fear that protecting their self-interests will result in rejection or retaliation. Here, instead of engaging in repair, opposite actions to reduce guilt and shame involve doing what one feels guilty or ashamed of over and over (e.g., learning to say no without excessive apologizing, guilt, or shame).

Sadness or Depression

Therapists explain that the natural behavior in response to despondency is to withdraw, becoming inactive and lethargic. Effective treatments for depression involve clients doing the opposite of these behaviors, such as getting out and being active, approaching, and doing things that make them feel competent and confident. This involves socializing with others, scheduling and getting involved in activities, and so forth.

The trap that many clients fall into, especially with the emotion of depression, is wanting to feel happier and more motivated before making a behavioral change, saying to themselves, "I want to feel like going out and being with friends first, and then I'll do it." Point out how this strategy backfires when clients act on what the emotion urges them to do, such as an urge to withdraw when depressed. With the emotion strengthened, clients are further ensnared in their depression.

Therapists might find it useful to emphasize that starting an opposite action behavior, such as exercise, especially for clients who are depressed, may not help them feel better immediately and may, in fact, make them feel worse. As discussed, this is what would be expected. Therapists can reassure clients that opposite behaviors do communicate a new and different message to the brain and that their brains *are* processing these but that time is required to translate these messages into emotional changes. One may not feel at all like socializing and being with others but must act "opposite" so that, slowly, positive emotional changes will follow. In summary, to change the emotion of sadness, clients must do the opposite of this emotion's action urge and become active.

Anger

The natural behavior associated with anger is to attack and hurt others. To change or reduce anger, therefore, clients must do the opposite. This may involve "taking a break" from the person a client is angry at (if she or he feels unable to communicate with that person without attacking) until she or he cools off. Acting Opposite may also involve doing something kind for the other person or putting oneself in the other person's shoes. Similar to avoiding reparations when feeling guilty, many clients are unwilling to act opposite to their anger out of the belief that being kind or having empathy for the other person would mean admitting to wrongdoing or necessitate judging oneself as bad.

It may be useful to emphasize that clients are choosing to change their anger, as well as their expressions of anger, only in cases in which that emotion is destructive and ineffective for achieving their goals. Remind clients that anger (or any emotion), whether justified or not, is valid. Past experiences may have understandably influenced clients to feel as they do. One of the key functions of anger may be to communicate to oneself that one has a right to be angry. However, if clients decide that it is not useful or effective for them to be angry to this degree, they may choose to act opposite even though the anger is valid. Therapists should make sure that clients do not mistake Acting Opposite for blocking, masking, or overdramatizing emotions.

Instead of outright anger, many clients may be more familiar with experiencing chronic irritability. This irritability may be justified but still not effective, as it can become self-perpetuating, leading others to be irritable in return and thus maintaining the emotion. Acting Opposite means accepting the irritability and its validity while choosing to act opposite to be more effective, such as by using gentle words or a light tone.

Why Binge Eating (and Purging) Is Not Acting Opposite

Discuss with clients how binge eating or other problematic eating behaviors have been attempts, albeit maladaptive, to use behaviors to change their experience of distressing emotions. One reason that these behaviors do not work effectively is that they do not involve Acting Opposite to the Current Emotion. Rather, they are likely to be quite consistent with the emotion. For example, when clients feel angry, binge eating (and purging) can be an expression of aggression, even if they are not outwardly attacking anyone. When clients feel guilt or shame, the binge eating (and purging) may express the urge to attack and punish themselves. Because the binge eating (and purging) is more or less consistent with the current emotion, these numbing or escaping behaviors serve to prolong the emotion rather than change it.

Therapists express their sincere understanding that Acting Opposite to the Current Emotion is extremely difficult. But continuing to act as clients have been, such as by binge eating and/or purging, reinforces clients' negative emotions and has debilitating consequences related to the behavior itself. Acting Opposite is an incredibly powerful skill that will, in the long run, offer true help.

◎ **DISCUSSION POINT:** *"Consider how practicing the skill of Acting Opposite to the Current Emotion may replace your binge eating and other problem eating behaviors. When you are depressed, for example, what might be the effect of getting active instead of spending the day isolated and overeating and/or purging? How could you use opposite action when you are in the throes of capitulating and believe you have no option except to turn to food?"*

Therapists may wish to use the following experiential exercise to further illustrate the skill of Acting Opposite.

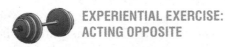

EXPERIENTIAL EXERCISE:
ACTING OPPOSITE

"Sit up straight, letting the chair fully support you. Take several deep, flowing breaths in and out. Find a place for your eyes to focus. Then bring to mind a recent situation in which you felt a strong negative emotion. Think about your reaction. Was it consistent with your emotion? If so, what was the effect? For example, perhaps you were depressed and you stayed in bed, or you were feeling hopeless and overweight and started binge eating, or were angry and started yelling? Now, take a moment to imagine that recent situation, validating the emotion but choosing to act the opposite. Try to consider how you may feel different as a result."

 DISCUSSION POINT: *"Can you describe what you imagined and how Acting Opposite affected your feelings?"*

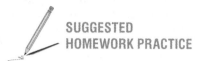

SUGGESTED
HOMEWORK PRACTICE

Remind clients that practicing the skills of observing and describing one's current emotion (e.g., using worksheets similar to Appendix 5.5) are essential to using the skill of opposite action. Unless one first accepts what she or he is feeling, she or he cannot become aware of what actions would be opposite nor when taking such actions would be effective. For example, observing and describing and increasing awareness of one's interpretations of events and body language associated with certain emotions may enable one to consider which opposite action to take to change ineffective emotions.

1. Therapists instruct clients to practice observing and describing a current emotion and to complete the homework sheet (e.g., Appendix 5.5).

2. Therapists instruct clients to think of ways to act opposite to their current emotion when wanting to reduce or change their current emotional experience and to write (e.g., at the bottom of Appendix 5.6) about what opposite actions were chosen. Ideally, clients should practice Acting Opposite at least three times prior to the next session.

MYTHS ABOUT EMOTIONS

The purpose of this section is to help clients challenge common myths about emotions. The Linehan Skills Manual Handout (1993b, p. 136), gives several examples of such myths: "There is a right way to feel in every situation"; "Negative feelings are bad and destructive"; and "If others do not approve of my feelings, I obviously shouldn't feel as I do."

Ask clients to generate their own myths about emotion, perhaps the myths that seem most linked with their binge eating (and purging) or myths they wrestle with when practicing the Emotion Regulation skills. Suggest that clients take 5 minutes or so and write down their challenges to these myths.

A typical emotion myth described by clients with binge eating (and purging) behaviors is "I won't be able to stand feeling this [emotion]." Therapists may wish to play devil's advocate (using a playful tone) in helping struggling clients to challenge this myth, such as by replying, "Oh my gosh, yes, I can see that this emotion is just killing you. Maybe we should get help, maybe call 911." Taking a devil's advocate position in this situation may make it more likely that the client shifts to a more dialectical view to effectively challenge her or his emotion myths (e.g.,

"Well, it's not going to kill me, and actually I have been able to stand it. I'm hoping with my new bag of tricks I'll be able to manage these upsetting emotions more effectively").

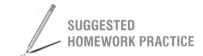

SUGGESTED HOMEWORK PRACTICE

1. Therapists instruct clients to review their emotion myths and challenges before the next session.

2. Therapists instruct clients to increase their awareness of any other emotion myths they hold that may not be effective. Are these related to the client's urges to binge eat (and purge)?

List of Emotion Regulation Skills

- Mindfulness of Your Current Emotion

- Loving Your Emotions

- Reducing Vulnerability to Emotion Mind

- Building Positive Experiences

- Mindfulness of Positive Experiences

- Opposite-to-Emotion Action

Model for Describing Emotions

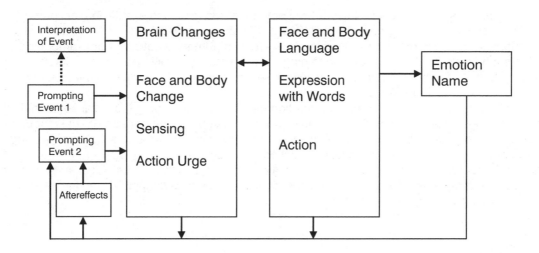

Primary Emotions and Secondary Reactions Homework Sheet

Primary emotions involve your initial, gut-level emotional responses to events. Typical primary emotions are love, joy, interest/excitement, fear, anger, and sadness. Primary thoughts, sensations, and behaviors are frequently associated with primary emotions. For example, a feeling such as excitement about an upcoming vacation may typically be accompanied by certain *thoughts* (e.g., "I can hardly wait for tomorrow!"), *sensations* (e.g., "butterflies in the stomach"), and *behaviors* (e.g., smiling).

Secondary reactions to the primary emotion usually involve judging the initial emotional response. The consequence of this evaluative judgment is that the primary emotional response is interrupted or halted, being replaced by secondary reactions. For example, in the preceding illustration, a secondary reaction to feeling excited might be the feeling of guilt, such as the thought "I shouldn't be feeling so happy about vacation with my mother being ill; instead of going I should spend my time off with her," and sensations, such as experiencing a knot in the pit of your stomach, slumping over, and so forth.

Instructions:

In the following space, write about at least one instance in which you noticed secondary reactions to your primary emotions. Be detailed in your description, both of the primary emotion (with its associated thoughts, behaviors, and sensations) and the secondary reactions. What were the consequences of your secondary reactions—did you feel worse? Write about what you think reinforces the secondary reactions.

Synopsis of Ways to Describe Emotions

Emotions	Love	Joy	Sadness	Anger	Fear
Synonyms	Affection Caring Arousal Compassion Kindness Warmth	Happiness Enjoyment Relief Amusement Hope Cheerfulness	Grief Misery Disappointment Hopelessness Depression Hurt Loneliness	Annoyance Bitterness Frustration Grouchiness Grumpiness Irritation	Anxiety Nervousness Being overwhelmed Panic Worry Tension
Prompting Events	Having special experience Having fun Being with someone	Feeling loved Being successful Desirable outcome Praise	Loss Separation Rejection Being disapproved of Being powerless/helpless	Being threatened Loss of respect Physical or emotional pain Not getting what you want out of a situation or person	Being threatened Novel situations Performing in front of others
Interpretations	"Someone loves me" "I'm good at this"	Interpreting joyful events as pleasurable	Seeing things as hopeless Thinking "I'm worthless"	"Things aren't fair"/"Things should be otherwise" (judgments)	"I'll get hurt" "I'm going to embarrass myself/fail" "They'll reject me"
Biological Changes and Experiences	Fast heartbeat Feeling self-confident Feeling happy	Feeling giggly, peaceful, calm Face flushing	Feeling tired Emptiness, hollowness in your chest Breathlessness	Feeling hot Face flushing Body rigid Jaws clenched Feeling out of control	Breathlessness Fast heart rate Clammy hands Muscle tension Nausea Butterflies in stomach
Expressions and Actions	Saying "I love …" Laughter Smiling Eye contact	Smiling Glowing Acting silly Excitement in voice Chattiness Being bouncy	Avoidance Acting helpless Moping Being inactive Slumping Crying	Clenched hands Face flushed Physical or verbal attack Frowning	Fleeing Avoiding Freezing Shaking
Aftereffects	Remembering other times feeling love Being positive Believing in myself	Being positive Being friendly and helpful Coping with worry Anticipating positive things	Negative outlook Blame, criticism Remembering being sad Hopelessness Numbness	Attention narrowing Rumination Feeling numb	Attention narrowing Hypervigilance to threat Daze/numbness Losing control Rumination
Secondary Emotions	Joy Contentment Sadness Shame Grief Anger Hatred	Love Loneliness Shame Guilt Embarrassment	Anger Shame Fear	Shame Fear Guilt	Anger Shame

Observing and Describing Emotions Homework Sheet

EMOTION NAME(S)   **Intensity** (0–100)

PROMPTING EVENT for emotion (who, what, when, where):

INTERPRETATIONS (beliefs, assumptions, appraisals) of situation:

BODY CHANGES and SENSING: What am I feeling in my body?

BODY LANGUAGE: What is my facial expression? Posture? Gestures?

ACTION URGES: What do I feel like doing? What do I want to say?

What **I SAID or DID** in the situation (Be specific):

What **AFTEREFFECTS** does the emotion have on me (state of mind, other emotions, thoughts, etc.)?

FUNCTION OF EMOTION:

Steps for Reducing Painful Emotions Homework Sheet

For each Emotion Regulation skill, check whether you used it during the week and describe what you did. Write on back of page if you need more room.

REDUCED VULNERABILITY TO EMOTION MIND: Treated physical illness? _____

Balanced eating? _____

Avoided mood-altering drugs? _____

Balanced sleep? _____

Exercised? _____

Practiced mastery? _____

INCREASED POSITIVE EVENTS

Increased daily pleasant activities (circle): M T W TH F S SUN   (Describe)

LONG-TERM GOALS worked on:

ATTENDED TO RELATIONSHIPS:

AVOIDED AVOIDING (Describe):

MINDFULNESS OF POSITIVE EXPERIENCES THAT OCCURRED

_____ Focused (and refocused) attention on positive experiences?

_____ Distracted from worries about positive experience?

MINDFULNESS OF THE CURRENT EMOTION

_____ Observed the emotion?   _____ Remembered:

_____ Experienced the emotion?   Not to act on emotion?

Times I've felt different?

OPPOSITE ACTION: How did I act opposite to the current emotion?

Adult Pleasant Events Schedule (Abbreviated)

1. Soaking in a bathtub
2. Going on vacation
3. Relaxing
4. Going to a movie in the beginning of the week
5. Laughing
6. Lying in the sun
7. Flying kites
8. Going to a party
9. Arranging flowers
10. Reading fiction
11. Gardening
12. Going hiking

CHAPTER 6

Distress Tolerance Skills

The aim of teaching Distress Tolerance skills is to equip clients with a variety of strategies to use *in the present moment* when they are experiencing pain, difficulty, or distress that cannot be changed right away. Essentially, Distress Tolerance skills are designed to teach clients how to bear pain skillfully. The idea is that everyone inevitably has to face pain and difficulty that is not within his or her control (e.g., natural disasters, illness, death of loved ones). At these times, it is critical to avoid making matters worse and to refrain from reacting in unskillful ways (e.g., binge eating, substance use) that can increase the pain and suffering. Although what is happening may be beyond one's control, one *can* choose to respond skillfully until things change. That is, eventually things will change (circumstances, emotions, etc., don't last forever), and using Distress Tolerance skills in the interim will put one in a better position when and if something *can* be done to improve things. At the heart of the Distress Tolerance skills is learning to develop patience, tolerance, and equanimity (nonreaction) in the face of difficulty that cannot be changed right away.

There are two different sets of Distress Tolerance skills: skills for Accepting Reality and Crisis Survival skills. *Skills for Accepting Reality* will enable the client to accept life as it is in the moment and cope with painful situations that cannot currently be changed. Specific skills include Observing Your Breath, Awareness Exercises, Half-Smiling, and Radical Acceptance (see Appendix 6.1). *Crisis Survival skills* are designed to facilitate the client's ability to bear short-term painful situations. Their aim is to help clients "carry on" and remain functional without resorting to behaviors that make things worse. Specific skills include Distracting, Self-Soothing, Improving the Moment, and Thinking of Pros and Cons (see Appendix 6.1).

Underlying the Acceptance of Reality skills is the notion that accepting, facing, and tolerating reality puts one in a stronger position to cope skillfully in the world, whereas trying to deny, fight, or avoid reality undermines coping and increases suffering. That is, acceptance encourages awareness such that understanding and compassion are more possible. Fighting, denying, or avoiding painful feelings decreases awareness and engages one in a struggle that therefore is not fully understood, increasing the likelihood of further suffering. Living skillfully involves accepting that pain and distress cannot be entirely avoided.

It is important to clarify that acceptance of reality does not imply approval of reality. Acceptance is not about approval or disapproval but involves simply acknowledging reality as it is rather than denying it. Clients can simultaneously accept reality and not like or not approve of it. As therapists acknowledge, things one likes are often easier to accept. The struggle is usually in coping with things one dislikes.

Crisis Survival skills are designed to provide clients with specific strategies to use when they are overwhelmed, feel unable or unwilling to accept the situation they are in, and/or cannot seem to locate their Wise Mind. Crisis Survival skills allow one to obtain much-needed momentary relief and a temporary break from overwhelming emotions so that, when returning to handling the crisis situation, one can do so in a different state of mind.

In summary, Distress Tolerance skills are aimed at helping clients learn to bear pain skillfully. By using Distress Tolerance skills to tolerate painful emotions when called for in that moment, clients can, paradoxically, *reduce* the intensity and duration of pain and suffering and *enhance* a feeling of mastery by using skillful means and wise responding. It is important that therapists highlight how Distress Tolerance skills are linked to the client's goals of stopping binge eating (and/or purging).

DISCUSSION POINT: *"What are your reactions to this material and its aims of teaching you to get through a difficult situation without making things worse, as well as how to survive a crisis when the situation cannot be changed right away? Can you think of times when trying to avoid pain led to more problems than it solved? How has binge eating or purging been used to avoid pain? How effective has it been, especially when viewed over the long run?"*

DISCUSSION POINT: *"Can you think of times when you needed to distract yourself or put your pain on the 'back burner' because it was not an appropriate time to work on changing or figuring out or resolving your painful emotions?"*

Therapists emphasize here that the distracting from or setting aside of one's pain is skillful. The purpose is to come back to it when the timing might be better. Also, the stepping back permits a calmer perspective. This is not denying or avoiding. Therapists might use the following story, or one from personal or clinical experience, to illustrate the potential consequences of attempting to deny reality and avoid pain.

ILLUSTRATIVE EXAMPLE
OF ATTEMPTING TO DENY REALITY AND AVOID PAIN

"A client in her 20s was denying her feelings about a relationship in an attempt to avoid the pain of ending it and experiencing loss. She didn't want to truly admit to herself how angry, hurt, and invalidated she felt. By avoiding her feelings and refusing to accept that the relationship was not working for her, she prolonged her suffering and stayed in the relationship for a year longer than was in her best interests. Looking back on this in later years, she realized that denying the reality meant enduring an additional year of this painful relationship and produced more pain than would have been the case if she had left when she knew it was time. If she had accepted the reality of her emotions and the pain of the situation a year prior, these emotions would have functioned to help her change the situation and end the relationship."

DISCUSSION POINT: *"Can you think of times when you accepted painful feelings? What was that experience of acceptance like for you? What can you recall about the consequences of accepting rather than fighting your experience?"*

OBSERVING YOUR BREATH

A useful skill that facilitates accepting reality is learning to be in the moment, one breath at a time. Breathing is something clients always have available to them. As therapists point out, no additional materials are needed. The skill of Observing Your Breath is designed to help center yourself or focus yourself on a single object in order to settle or calm the mind. This is a particularly useful skill to employ when you are agitated, overwhelmed, distracted, and/or preoccupied. Observing Your Breath can help to access the Wise Mind.

There are many variations and examples of this skill. For example, clients might practice observing their breath when listening to music, when walking, when carrying on a conversation, and so forth (see Linehan, 1993b, Distress Tolerance Handout 2, pp. 170–171).

Therapists may wish to use the following script, modifying it as needed, to lead clients in the experiential exercise of counting breaths as an example of Observing Your Breath.

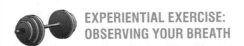

EXPERIENTIAL EXERCISE:
OBSERVING YOUR BREATH

"Get into a comfortable position with your feet on the floor, head and spine straight, and breathe in and out from your diaphragm, taking slow, deep, rhythmic breaths. Choose a spot on which to focus your eyes, or gently close them. Bring your attention to your breath coming in and going out. Try to settle your body, keeping the breath in mind as your anchor. As you inhale, be aware that you are inhaling. When you exhale, be aware that you are exhaling. If you are feeling anxious or experiencing some discomfort as you breathe, just note this and gently turn your mind to breathing in and out. Make your breathing as comfortable as possible. If breathing from your diaphragm is not comfortable for you, find a spot to focus the breath that is comfortable for you. Now, as you inhale, begin counting by saying: 'I am inhaling ... one.' Then, as you slowly exhale, say: 'I am exhaling ... one.' Keep counting—'I am inhaling ... two' ... 'I am exhaling ... two'—until you reach ten. When at ten, return to counting with one. Practice keeping your mind fully engaged in the breathing. Any time your mind wanders, just bring it back to the exercise and begin again at one."

 DISCUSSION POINT: *"What was your experience with the exercise? Did the practice help in attending to and accepting the moment?"*

Therapists are advised to underscore the importance of practice. Observing Your Breath can be practiced at various points throughout the day. Five or ten minutes of practice three or four times a day will pay off over time and strengthen one's ability to use this skill in times of stress. Observing Your Breath can be done in a variety of contexts, including those daily struggles, annoying situations, and minicrises that one seems to continually confront. Additionally, clients can use the skill of Observing Your Breath at times when they feel the urge to do something unskillful or destructive (e.g., reaching for something to eat) in response to unpleasant feelings they are having about a particular situation (e.g., not wanting to accept that heavy traffic will make them 15 minutes late). Not every challenge can be avoided. If a person tries to respond to and change every stressful thing in his or her life, he or she is likely to end up frustrated and plain worn out. This exhaustion can, in turn, make one more vulnerable to urges to turn to food. Practicing the skill of Observing Your Breath on a daily basis can fortify a client's ability to nonreactively accept the reality of her or his situation.

 DISCUSSION POINT: *"Are you experiencing a distressing situation in your life right now? If so, could you imagine applying the Observe Your Breath skill to that situation?"*

Therapists may want to conduct the following experiential exercise to illustrate applying the skill of Observing Your Breath.

 EXPERIENTIAL EXERCISE:
COUNTING YOUR BREATHS WHEN EXPERIENCING DISTRESS

"Sit comfortably in your chair with an upright but not rigid posture and begin to focus on your breathing. Choose a focus point for your eyes or gently close them. Bring your full attention to breathing in and out as comfortably as you can. Let your mind settle as best you can, keeping your attention on your breathing. Now bring a distressing situation to mind. See yourself in the situation, picturing what you are doing, saying, and feeling. Then see yourself in the situation using the skill of Observing Your Breath. See yourself maintaining a focus on breathing despite the reality of the distressing situation. See yourself being patient with the breath, nonreactive, acknowledging what is happening but not fighting what is. Remember that you don't have to *do* anything in this moment to alter what is, and that accepting the situation is not the same as approving it. Just stay with observing your inhalations and exhalations and do not get pulled away or distracted by thoughts or feelings regardless of how compelling they are. Stay with the breath as your center even as you are aware of the distress 'at the edges.' Observing any accompanying thoughts or feelings is a part of Observing Your Breath. Practice till you get to a count of ten. Then end the exercise."

DISCUSSION POINT: *"What were your experiences when practicing Observing Your Breath? Did your distress lessen, intensify, or stay the same? Can you imagine employing this skill? When might it be useful to you to do so? What result would you hope to achieve?"*

DISCUSSION POINT: *"What are your reactions to the idea that there does not have to be a resolution to your distressing situation and that, indeed, there is not always a pain-free solution available to many of life's biggest challenges? What do you think the effect would be of finding out you can survive and tolerate the distress you are experiencing without making it worse?"*

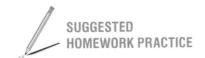

SUGGESTED HOMEWORK PRACTICE

Therapists should encourage clients to remember as they practice these skills that truly learning to accept the moment and tolerate whatever difficult feelings are present should help lessen the intensity of clients' urges to block or change their feelings through binge eating and/or purging.

1. Therapists instruct clients to practice an Observing Your Breath exercise each day. This might involve counting their breaths, observing their breath when listening to music, observing their breath when walking, or observing their breath when carrying on a conversation.

2. Therapists encourage clients to discover which is their favorite.

HALF-SMILING

The skill of Half-Smiling is a very powerful one. For many clients it becomes a favorite. The skill's aim is to facilitate clients' inner acceptance by having them adopt an outer facial expression of acceptance—the half-smile. When one's facial muscles are tight or one's jaw is set, it is very difficult to accept something. The outer tightness is incompatible with an accepting inner attitude. With Half-Smiling, the muscles of the face are relaxed. By adopting a half-smile—a serene, accepting smile—clients increase their chances of experiencing internal acceptance.

Experimental evidence shows that one's facial expression communicates with one's brain. We are accustomed to thinking about our brains communicating with our faces; we internally experience an emotion (e.g., sadness, happiness) that sends a signal to our faces (e.g., to frown, to smile). Yet there is evidence that the communication also works in the other direction. For example, in one study (e.g., Laird, 1974), participants were asked to place their facial muscles in various positions.

The positions were added slowly and were so out of sequence that the participants did not know what position their faces were in. Participants whose outer expressions were angry were more likely to experience anger inwardly, those whose outer expressions were sad were more likely to experience sadness inwardly, and so forth. That is, the research found that one's outer facial expressions communicate with and give feedback to one's brain.

Half-Smiling is not intended to be used to avoid or deny one's experience. One employs Half-Smiling with the knowledge that it is skillful to do so under the circumstances. While fully aware of the myriad experiences one may be having, one chooses to promote the experience of acceptance by adopting a half-smile. This skill helps clients to access their Wise Mind, which accepts reality skillfully with awareness but without judgment. Clients need not completely understand the source or basis of their distress in choosing to practice the Half-Smiling skill. Wise responding involves tolerating their experience.

Clients are taught how to practice the skill of Half-Smiling. The following experiential exercise can be used, modifying the script as needed.

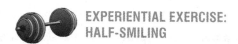

EXPERIENTIAL EXERCISE: HALF-SMILING

"Begin by putting your face in a neutral position. If it helps, close your eyes, though this is not required. From the neutral face, make a very angry face, one you'd make if you were really infuriated. If you are having difficulty, try to imagine a situation in which you were absolutely livid or 'fit to be tied.' As your face is in this position, pay attention to your inner experience. Now change your expression to the neutral face again, taking several deep breaths from your diaphragm. Now, create the facial expression you make when you are afraid or highly anxious—a face of fear. If needed, think of a time when you were really and truly afraid. Once again, pay attention to your inner experience as you make the facial expression of fear.

"Now, place your facial muscles in a neutral position again, taking several deep diaphragmatic breaths. Now, adopt a sad expression, perhaps one that is grief stricken. Pay attention to the inner experience accompanying this facial expression. Then, come back to the neutral face, taking a few moments.

"Now, turn the corners of your mouth up very slightly into a half-smile. It is important to remember that when you half-smile, your face is completely relaxed. Imagine any tension fading away, as if a cool iron were smoothing the muscles of your face, neck, and shoulders, helping them to relax. Your forehead, eyes, cheeks, and jaw muscles are just 'hanging' on your face. Ever so slightly, turn up the corners of your lips toward your ears. It's just a slight upturn of the lips, not really a smile, but still perceptibly different from the neutral face. This half-smile is not a tense expression, nor is it a grin or a smirk. Perhaps it might help to think of the Mona Lisa's smile. Stay with that position, and pay attention to your internal experience."

DISCUSSION POINT: *"What did you notice about your inner experiences when you adopted the different outer facial expressions? What was your experience of the half-smile? Did you notice a greater feeling of being open to acceptance?"*

If helpful, emphasize the point made earlier that in choosing to put on a half-smile, clients are not masking, denying, or hiding their emotions. Half-Smiling involves acknowledgment of whatever one's experience is, followed by the decision to call up a different experience. The client is choosing to facilitate inner acceptance by placing her or his facial muscles into an accepting, relaxed pattern.

Therapists remind clients of the Model for Describing Emotions (Chapter 5, Appendix 5.2). According to that model, a stimulus causes the brain to react, triggering certain neurochemical and facial muscle changes. Half-Smiling changes the emotional experience by changing the client's facial expression. This feedback changes the client's brain chemistry. Compared with some of the other acceptance skills that clients will be taught, which involve *thinking* about one's experience differently, adopting a half-smile is a *physical* behavior that clients can employ as a catalyst for change.

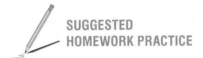

SUGGESTED HOMEWORK PRACTICE

1. Therapists instruct clients to list situations that would be useful for practicing Half-Smiling—situations in which they cannot change the reality of their circumstances and find it difficult to achieve acceptance (e.g., waiting in line, being stuck in traffic, having one's bus, train, or plane delayed).

2. Therapists encourage clients to practice Half-Smiling at least once a day to gain familiarity with this new skill. Suggest that clients practice this skill when they experience an urge to binge and/or purge.

GUIDELINES FOR ACCEPTING REALITY: AWARENESS EXERCISES

The purpose of the Awareness Exercises is to practice keeping one's attention focused in the current moment, fully aware and present. Awareness Exercises help cultivate the ability to be aware of each moment, and practicing these skills strengthens awareness and acceptance in the moment so as to develop a more accepting state of mind. Emphasize that learning and strengthening the ability to accept reality as it is, without making it worse with behaviors such as binge eating and/or purging, is extremely valuable. If well practiced, these skills can be highly cherished tools for helping one accept and tolerate the reality of very tough times. Acceptance is not intended to include acceptance of the state of things as they are for eternity but acceptance of how things are in the moment. Thus the emphasis with acceptance is on awareness of the current moment.

It is best to practice these or any new skills and to build one's "Awareness" muscle by selecting relatively simple tasks and situations, as opposed to complicated emotional situations, as one's focus. The Awareness Exercises involve practicing being mindful of tasks such as making tea or coffee or brushing one's teeth rather than solving complex equations or preparing a tax return. It is best to practice awareness of simple daily activities at the outset. Other ideas for experiential exercises include awareness while washing dishes, walking slowly in a circle, taking a slow-motion bath, applying lotion, and so forth.

The Awareness Exercises involve utilization of the core Mindfulness skills, or the ability to nonjudgmentally participate with awareness. Many of these exercises, including Observing Your Breath, Half-Smiling, and Awareness, are adapted from the book *The Miracle of Mindfulness: A Manual of Meditation* by the Zen master Thich Nhat Hanh (1999). Clients who would like further reading on mindfulness and the acceptance of reality exercises are referred to this book.

The following short experiential exercise can be used to help clients practice awareness, modifying the script as needed.

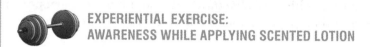

EXPERIENTIAL EXERCISE:
AWARENESS WHILE APPLYING SCENTED LOTION

"Lavender-scented lotion is being passed around. Practice being aware and fully in the moment as you smooth the lotion on your hands and skin. The idea is to participate with awareness, focusing your attention on just the moment you are in."

DISCUSSION POINT: *"What was that like? Were you able to be fully present for your experience, or did you find your mind wandering off? Do you think you are usually present for these types of everyday experiences, or are you on automatic pilot? How do you think these awareness exercises could help facilitate emotional acceptance and disrupt the path to binge eating, purging, or mindless eating?"*

RADICAL ACCEPTANCE

Radical Acceptance involves letting go of fighting reality through accepting from deep within oneself, at the core of one's being. The word "radical" is Latin for "root." In other words, Radical Acceptance involves accepting reality at its root or core. It is not a superficial type of acceptance. Rather, it is characterized by the serenity prayer, which, as clients may know, says, "Grant me the serenity to accept the things I cannot change, the courage to change the things I can, and the wisdom to know the difference." Ultimately, Radical Acceptance involves accepting the way things are; there are circumstances that cause pain and that one cannot change; one must accept the resulting pain. Additionally, Radical Acceptance is accepting that one must change the things that one can and accept the complicated, tough, and painful feelings about the situation, as well as any that may arise as a consequence of making changes.

Radical Acceptance can be a powerful tool for clients as they struggle to change the things they can (i.e., binge eating, purging, and other maladaptive eating behaviors). Practicing Radical Acceptance can be very helpful for clients who experience bodily symptoms after stopping compensatory behaviors (e.g., edema, or swelling, after cessation of laxative abuse). Practicing Radical Acceptance would involve accepting both the physical and psychological discomforts of a Wise Mind decision to change.

The following exercise can be used to introduce clients to the concept of Radical Acceptance, modifying as needed.

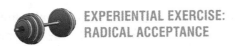

EXPERIENTIAL EXERCISE:
RADICAL ACCEPTANCE

"Sit up straight in your chair, feet on the floor, with your hands resting comfortably. Pick a place to focus your eyes (or gently close them) and take a moment to focus your mind on your breath. Now, think back to a time in your life when you were given bad news, something that at first you didn't accept. [Pause] Perhaps it was a loss of some sort, or a death. Remember what you felt at the time. What were your initial emotions? Was your tendency to avoid your feelings or deny the reality of what was happening? [Pause] Now, think about when you were able to acknowledge what had happened and accept the reality of the situation. Describe the difference between those two experiences—your nonacceptance of the reality of the situation and your acceptance of the situation. Take a moment now to practice Radical Acceptance of the pain you experienced as a consequence of the situation you brought to mind. Take five deep, flowing breaths, slowly opening your eyes if you had them closed, as we end the exercise."

 DISCUSSION POINT: *"What did you notice about the two experiences—when you did not accept the reality of the situation and when you did accept it?"*

Emphasize that acceptance is not the same thing as resignation or passivity. Indeed, not only is acceptance not antithetical or contrary to change, but acceptance is required for change, for being able to act. Clients must first accept the reality of a situation before they can act to change it. Not accepting a situation leaves one stuck.

Following is a clinical example used in our groups to make the preceding point regarding the necessity of accepting something in order to bring about change.

ILLUSTRATIVE EXAMPLE:
ACCEPTANCE IS NOT PASSIVITY

"Imagine the terrible situation of a child being molested by a babysitter. For many people, if this happened to their child or to a child they knew, the tendency would be to deny the situation, at least at first, because the reality feels too painful to face. But one has to at least face up to the reality of the situation in order to act—for example, informing the authorities or removing the child to a safe situation.

"Or think about the example of binge eating [and purging]. If you deny or continually avoid facing the truth that you are eating in a disordered way or try to ignore how hurtful and disruptive this behavior is to your life, does this increase or decrease the likelihood that you will remain stuck in the behavior?

"In other words, acceptance is a choice. You can live facing reality or you can ignore reality. Radical Acceptance is making the choice to accept the moment, whatever it is, and thus accept the pain. Paradoxically, Radical Acceptance may transform your experience. Fighting painful feelings and refusing to accept that pain is an inevitable part of life can interfere with reducing pain and instead may lead to prolonging pain and suffering."

It is useful to acknowledge the impulse clients may experience to accept something while holding onto a secret hope that doing so will mean that they will not have to experience pain. Therapists will want to make clear that acceptance is not an internal bargaining chip; clients cannot say "OK, I'll accept this intense disappointment, but the deal is that the disappointment will automatically go away." When clients are trying to use acceptance as a technique to create change, they are not really accepting. Clients are not practicing accepting the reality from deep within.

Therapists should also point out that acceptance does not mean having to give up hope that a situation will improve or that one's pain will decrease. Clients can hope for these changes but should not necessarily expect use of Radical Acceptance to make them feel better.

Suffering Is the Nonacceptance of Pain

Therapists define suffering as the struggle to keep pain out of awareness. In other words, suffering is pain *plus* the nonacceptance of pain. The struggle to escape or deny pain ensures that clients remains engaged in the effort not to accept things as they are. This, as a result, creates suffering. Being stuck fighting reality and not accepting pain generates and maintains suffering.

The good news about the skill of Radical Acceptance, as therapists should describe, is that it can transform the struggle of suffering into the experience of this current moment's pain. It cannot be overemphasized that acceptance does not mean that pain goes away. But acceptance means that one does not suffer as much. Pain may be unavoidable, but when the client accepts it, she or he is dealing only with the pain rather than with the pain *plus* the nonacceptance of that pain.

 DISCUSSION POINT: *"Can you think of examples from your life in which you experienced Radical Acceptance?"*

Therapists may find the following experiential exercise useful in helping clients practice Radical Acceptance, modifying as needed.

 EXPERIENTIAL EXERCISE:
ACCEPTING THE PAIN OF A CURRENT SITUATION

"Sit comfortably in your chairs, choosing a place for your eyes to focus. Bring to mind something you are not accepting now. Perhaps there is some situation, some aspect of your reality that you are resisting or fighting. As you bring that thing to mind, practice accepting it, practicing acknowledging it. You are practicing accepting the reality of the situation. This acceptance may mean acknowledging that this is a situation you can do nothing about, at least for the moment. Or the acceptance may mean acknowledging that there is something that you can do, that there are changes you must make. Practice acceptance right now of whatever you might be fighting, denying, or resisting.

"Remember as you practice the acceptance that you are acknowledging reality. If a situation has caused you to become hurt, Radical Acceptance means accepting this pain as a consequence of that situation, as a reality that has occurred. This means accepting it as just what is. Think about how we accept gravity. We do not feel we have to like it or approve of it. But we are able to accept that objects fall as a consequence of gravitational forces. Radically accepting gravity allows us to let go of struggling against such realities. We do not have to be 'OK' with gravity to radically accept it, nor must we remain passive."

Turning the Mind

The first step toward Radical Acceptance is being aware that you have the choice to accept. When you notice yourself turning away from acceptance, it is possible to turn your mind back to the path of acceptance. Turning the Mind is the opposite of capitulating. Capitulating is refusing to see any path but one. It is saying, for example, "I have no other options. The only thing I can do here is use food." Capitulating closes off the path of acceptance, of the reality of the situation that just occurred, and involves rigidly staying on whatever maladaptive path one is on, refusing to even consider, let alone choose, another path.

Turning the Mind is the first step toward opening oneself up to another option. Clearly, simply acknowledging the existence of another path or bringing to clients' awareness that they have a choice does not mean that they will necessarily take that path. But clients are more likely to do so if they are aware that this option is there.

 DISCUSSION POINT: *"Can you give an example of a time when you recognized that there was another option than remaining caught in a struggle that was not effective?"*

Willingness and Willfulness

After one becomes aware of the choice to take the path of acceptance, Willingness is needed. Willingness is the state of doing what is necessary in each situation. It involves focusing on effectiveness, listening carefully to one's Wise Mind, acting from one's inner self. Willingness is allowing the awareness of a larger perspective, the awareness of a broader meaning to the things that are happening that one dislikes.

Willfulness is refusing to do what is needed in the situation or, metaphorically, sitting on one's hands when action is needed. Willfulness can mean giving up, or it can mean trying to fix every situation, refusing to tolerate the moment.

Willingness is making an agreement with oneself that one will accept reality and act skillfully as opposed to willfully refusing to deal with reality on its own terms.

The following illustrative example may be useful for clients in making the distinction between willingness and willfulness.

ILLUSTRATIVE EXAMPLE: WILLINGNESS AND WILLFULNESS

"Imagine that for months you had planned a very special outdoor garden party. As the event approaches, the forecast calls for rain. Willfulness would be denying the forecast, saying, 'No—it is *not* going to rain. I've been planning and planning. I don't have room for an indoor party, and this party is going to be outside and it won't rain.' Then, on the day of the party, it rains, and you're furious. Willfulness is refusing to go with reality on its own terms. Willingness, on the other hand, is deciding that the forecast may be accurate and making arrangements, even if you would rather not, to be able to move the party indoors if needed or renting tents so that your guests can still be comfortable if it rains.

"If life is like a card game, then you have a choice to play the hand that you have been dealt as skillfully as you can, being mindful of and accepting your cards. This is choosing willingness. Or you can throw your cards down and say, 'I'm not going to play. It's not fair.' That's willfulness."

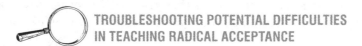 **DISCUSSION POINT:** *"Do you see binge eating and/or purging as being willful? Do you use food as a way of sitting on your hands when action is needed? Is it a way of giving up, trying to fix every situation, refusing to tolerate the moment? What are your thoughts?"*

TROUBLESHOOTING POTENTIAL DIFFICULTIES IN TEACHING RADICAL ACCEPTANCE

- *Example 1*: "Is Radical Acceptance the same thing as forgiveness?"

- *Potential therapist reply*: "Radical Acceptance should not be confused with forgiveness. Forgiveness is a choice, not a necessary outcome of Radical Acceptance. Practicing Radical Acceptance helps you honor your emotions (e.g., hurt, anger, resentment) and the fact that they are present. Once these emotions are acknowledged, you may choose to forgive by acting opposite to your emotions and to the action urges associated with them. Forgiveness comes easier to some than others. You may want to forgive if enduring these emotions interferes with your quality of life. When you've radically accepted your hurt and anger, you may be able to forgive if you develop a sense of compassion for the person who caused your pain. It's your choice whether you want to reach forgiveness."

- *Example 2*: "Why do I find it so hard to accept things even when it's in my best interest?"

- *Potential therapist reply*: "I know you're not sure, but has anything come to mind about what you think makes it difficult to take the first step of turning your mind toward acceptance? Perhaps these ideas might be helpful in triggering some thoughts. For some of us, what makes it hard is the fear that, if we are willing to accept things as they are, that means that we, our situation, or the problems we're struggling over will never change. If that rings true for you, it might be helpful to remind yourself that acceptance does not mean you are powerless or passive. It might also be helpful to think about how 'acceptance' is about accepting the way things are in this one moment, not all moments to come or moments that have passed. It also may help to reflect about what is effective for you in a situation. Sometimes we must accept that we must work to do what is needed in order to be effective—and that this includes dealing with reality the way it is."

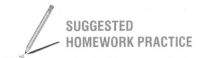

SUGGESTED HOMEWORK PRACTICE

Therapists instruct clients to practice Radical Acceptance (including Turning the Mind and Willingness) by spending some time each day purposefully focusing on this skill. Specifically, clients may find it helpful to keep track of how distressed they feel (on a scale of 1–100) prior to practicing Radical Acceptance and how distressed they feel afterward.

BURNING YOUR BRIDGES

Burning Your Bridges is another Radical Acceptance skill. It involves accepting, on a very deep level, that one is really never going to binge (and purge) again. Clients "burn" the binge eating (and purging) bridge so that this behavior is not an alternative. What is radical about this skill is that it involves saying, "Regardless of my experience, turning to food just won't be an option. There are other ways I am going to deal with whatever my experience is."

Therapists can point out that practicing Burning Your Bridges is similar to what people who stop smoking by going "cold turkey" do. These individuals make a pact that this will be their last cigarette. No matter what cravings or experiences arise, it is not an option for them to smoke. Burning Your Bridges involves Radical Acceptance of one's experiences. It may also mean that clients act to cut off all options to binge eat (and purge). In other words, clients may practice this skill by disposing of binge foods, by not engaging in certain situations that have repeatedly made them vulnerable to binge eating and purging, or by not engaging in those apparently irrelevant behaviors that almost always lead them, sooner or later, to misuse food.

The following experiential exercise can be used to further illustrate this skill, modifying the script as needed.

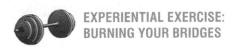

EXPERIENTIAL EXERCISE: BURNING YOUR BRIDGES

"Make yourself comfortable in your chair, with an erect posture, your head up straight, and your feet on the floor. Take several deep breaths from your diaphragm—choosing a place to focus your eyes. Now, imagine that you are on the coastline looking out at an island from the shore. This island is 'Binge Eating [and

Purging] Island.' Imagine what this island of binge eating [and purging] looks like. Next, picture the water separating you from the island filled with sharks, with the only way to reach the island being a bridge.

"Now, imagine placing a stick of dynamite on each slat of the bridge. It may be helpful to think about what the slats symbolize for you, such as the individual behaviors that make it possible for you to continue to reach Binge Eating [and Purging] Island. These might include your personal apparently irrelevant behaviors—for instance, hosting parties and not getting rid of leftovers or shopping when you're ravenous. Take time to identify those situations or apparently irrelevant behaviors that your Wise Mind knows end up, sooner or later, leading you to Binge Eating [and Purging] Island.

"Once you're safely back on shore, imagine detonating the dynamite. Visualize each slat of the bridge blowing up, one by one, until the whole bridge has exploded. You've now burned your bridge to Binge Eating [and Purging] Island. Binge eating [and purging] is not an option ever again. Take a moment to imagine being in a situation in which you feel an urge to binge or purge and looking back out to the island and saying, 'Oh, I've burned that bridge, it's just not an option.'"

 DISCUSSION POINT: *"What came to mind? How did it feel to imagine feeling an urge and knowing the bridge was blown up?"*

After teaching Burning Your Bridges, it is often a natural time to have clients recommit to stopping binge eating (and purging). The following sample script for leading clients through the recommitment exercise can be modified as needed.

 EXPERIENTIAL EXERCISE:
RECOMMITTING TO STOPPING BINGE EATING (AND PURGING)

"As was mentioned, people who make commitments to do something are more likely to be successful. So what we'd like you to do is to recommit, out loud, to the same commitment you made during the first session—to stop binge eating [and/or purging]. But now, as compared with then, you know so many more skills, and many of you already have stopped binge eating [and/or purging]. So this is taking it a bit further and fully committing yourself to never taking the bridge to binge eating [and/or purging] again. That path never worked for you. Avoiding your emotions and using food as a way of coping brought you to the point at which you came into this program. You had recognized that binge eating [and purging] was preventing you from building the quality of life you wanted and that you had to stop in order to build an authentic relationship with yourself and others and to feel that you were living up to your potential. Take a moment and get in touch with your Wise Mind and, if and when you're ready, recommit to stopping binge eating [and/or purging]."

 DISCUSSION POINT:
"What was that like for you?"

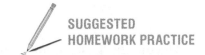

Therapists instruct clients to practice bringing up the image of Burning Your Bridges to binge eating (and purging) at least once a day. Using the homework sheet (Appendix 6.2), clients can write about their practice of this skill, including their thoughts and feelings about their use of it.

CRISIS SURVIVAL SKILLS

Introduction to Crisis Survival Skills

This next group of Distress Tolerance skills, the Crisis Survival skills, is introduced by explaining that these strategies are intended to help clients survive a crisis without making matters worse. Crisis Survival skills can be extremely useful for those painful events and emotions about which nothing can be done, at least not at the current moment.

According to the dictionary, a crisis is defined as a "turning point" in the course, a crucial time, stage, or event. In other words, a crisis is a time of danger or trouble whose outcome decides whether possible bad consequences will follow. The synonym for a crisis is an emergency.

Emphasize that a crisis can be a turning point in that the way clients handle it affects the outcome. Interestingly, as some clients may already know, the Chinese symbol for crisis is apparently the merging of two symbols—the symbol for danger and the symbol for opportunity. Put another way, a crisis entails both the danger that one can react to—thus potentially making the situation worse (e.g., by turning to binge eating)—as well as the opportunity to respond more adaptively. Not making matters worse may in and of itself be very affirming.

Remind clients of the point made earlier in the module: that the Crisis Survival skills should not be reserved for only the "big" crises in one's life. Crises exist in varying degrees of severity, the minicrises and the bigger ones. Furthermore, what one client defines as a crisis may not fit another's definition. These skills can be used for the daily minicrises that make a client's life more stressful.

When everything else the client is doing is not working for her or him, and it feels as though all her or his skills have gone out the window, the Crisis Survival strategies are the skills to try to practice. In other words, crises (both big and small) occur when one feels unable to accept one's situation, does not feel willing, and cannot seem to locate Wise Mind.

Therapists clarify that Crisis Survival skills are not intended to solve the crisis but to provide momentary relief so that when clients return to handling the crisis situation they can do so in a different state of mind. Caution clients that Crisis Survival skills are not meant to be overly used, as they can lose their effectiveness over time. In addition, they are not intended to be the only skills clients use, because these skills were not designed to and thus do not solve longer term problems. In other words, these are very valuable skills, but it is important that they be a *part* of the clients' repertoires of skills.

Overview of Crisis Survival Skills

Give an overview of the Crisis Survival skills that will be taught: Distraction skills, Self-Soothing skills, skills for Improving the Moment, and skills that help clients Think of the Pros and Cons of tolerating their distress. The reason for so many different types of skills is that surviving an emotional crisis takes a great deal of skill and effort. Different situations warrant the use of different skills. Having as many different Crisis Survival skills in one's toolbox as possible is an advantage because one can draw from them as needed.

Underscore the importance of maintaining an open mind while practicing these skills, as clients never know what exactly might be effective. Therapists make clear that, of course, the skills that will be mentioned are not an exhaustive list. Clients can add to it things that would be helpful to them. The one criterion for a Crisis Survival skill is that it helps the client survive the crisis without making things worse. It shouldn't be something that ends up allowing one to shoot oneself in the foot.

 DISCUSSION POINT:
"What are situations you need to 'survive' in your life right now?"

Distraction Skills

The purpose of these skills is to temporarily reduce clients' contact with emotional triggers or situations that are too overwhelming. Therapists explain that in such situations, clients need to refocus outside of themselves and outside of the situations they are in in order to give themselves a much-needed break. The idea is to interrupt the crisis long enough to reduce their tension, so that when the clients return to the crisis they are at least a little bit renewed or have a slightly different perspective.

One category of distraction skills involves distracting oneself with *activities*, such as exercise, hobbies, cleaning, going to events, calling and visiting with a friend, and so forth. Another category includes distracting by *contributing*. The idea here is that by contributing one gets in touch with a different experience from that of the current crisis. Many clients report this skill to be very useful to them. The contribution does not have to be a big one. It might involve saying hello to someone. Another type of distraction involves making *comparisons*. It can be helpful to think of others who are experiencing a worse situation or who are less fortunate. Therapists acknowledge that doing this can initially be a bit off-putting for some but that clients should try to keep open minds. Therapists might educate clients about research on the phenomenon of a "downward comparison" that suggests that comparing oneself with individuals worse off than oneself can improve one's mood. Reiterate that the reason so many skills are presented is to allow clients to find one or more that will work for them in a certain situation.

Another way to distract oneself is by bringing up *opposite emotions*. By becoming involved in something that will result in a different and positive emotion rather than an upsetting one, clients can distract themselves. Some suggestions include watching comedies (e.g., movies, TV shows), listening to soothing or uplifting music, reading a funny book—anything that will get clients involved in a different emotional experience.

Clients can also distract themselves through *pushing away*, or leaving the situation. If possible, this can entail physically removing oneself for a period, which can be incredibly helpful. If clients cannot leave physically, they might try "leaving" mentally—perhaps by envisioning boxing up the overwhelming situation or feelings and putting the box high on the shelf. Again, the purpose of this skill is to help clients take a temporary break.

Another means of distracting is the use of *other intense situations*. For example, clients might stand under a very hot shower, immerse their faces in ice water (many find this particularly effective at triggering a calming response), hold ice cubes in their hands, listen to very loud music, and so forth. Clients should be encouraged to do things that distract them from whatever the emotional trigger is so that they can experience something different.

It is important to remind clients to practice Crisis Survival skills One-Mindfully. These skills often will not work if clients are practicing a Crisis Survival skill while simultaneously thinking about the crisis.

⊚ **DISCUSSION POINT:** *"Do you have examples of times when you've distracted yourself? When did you? How well or not did it work? Are there other types of distractions that have not been mentioned that you do or have done in the past that are effective?"*

Self-Soothing Skills

When clients are emotionally overwhelmed, the thing for them to do is to comfort, nurture, and be gentle with themselves. Therapists might point out that clients would likely suggest this strategy to someone else undergoing a crisis, but, commonly, when people face crises themselves, kindness either does not come to mind or they are actively criticizing and berating themselves for experiencing the crisis and/or for not being able to resolve it. Yet having compassion for oneself is key.

The skill of Self-Soothing can be organized by the five senses to make it easier for clients to remember. When practicing self-soothing with *vision*, clients might buy a beautiful bouquet of flowers, light a candle, visit a museum filled with beautiful art, look at nature, and/or go out in the middle of the night to watch the stars.

When practicing this skill, clients should incorporate the Mindfulness skills, such as being mindful of each sight that passes in front of them. In other words, by putting themselves in the state of mind of acceptance, of being in just this one moment, clients may find it easier to get through a crisis without making it worse.

When clients self-soothe with *hearing*, they might try listening to beautiful, peaceful music, or they might practice paying attention to the sounds of nature around them, such as the chirping of birds and crickets. Clients might also hum a soothing song to themselves (e.g., a favorite tune or a lullaby). Therapists should emphasize that self-soothing music should not include music that triggers problem behaviors (e.g., music that one associates with binge eating and/or purging).

Self-soothing can also involve the client's sense of *smell*. Clients might use their favorite lotions or perfumes, light a scented candle, boil cinnamon, and/or mindfully breathe in the fresh smells of nature.

With some clients with eating disorders, self-soothing with *taste* will work well, but not with others. If a client decides to practice self-soothing with taste, using her or his Wise Mind to help decide, the practice should involve tasting and/or eating mindfully. Potential ways to practice might include having a soothing hot drink, such as a cup of flavorful tea, sucking on a piece of candy, treating oneself to a single portion of a tasty dessert, putting whipped cream on one's coffee, and so forth. Encourage clients to really taste and savor the food they are eating.

Clients choosing to practice self-soothing with *touch* might take a bubble bath, have a massage, treat themselves to a manicure or pedicure, pet their dogs or cats, soak their feet, put a cold compress on their foreheads, or cuddle under a soft or heated blanket.

 DISCUSSION POINT: *"Do you tend to ignore your sensations when in a crisis? Would these skills, designed to help you be gentle with yourself, be useful to you for everyday crises, as well as for especially difficult times?"*

 DISCUSSION POINT:
"Have you tried these types of things? Can you imagine doing so?"

Improving the Moment

The Crisis Survival skills of Improving the Moment are intended to help clients stay in just the moment they are in, making that moment more palatable than it would be otherwise. Although just that one moment is improved, clients may find that having this new experience breaks up the unrelenting nature of the crisis, helping them to survive the situation they are trying to bear without making things worse by engaging in self-destructive behaviors such as binge eating.

Improving the Moment with *imagery* includes visualizing relaxing scenes, imagining coping well, and so forth. Encourage clients by informing them how effective the use of imagery can be as a tool. Therapists must be careful, however, to remind clients that this skill can be particularly difficult to access during a crisis, particularly without prior experience. Therefore it is very important to gain practice using imagery during nonstressful periods.

Improving the Moment with *meaning* involves clients finding or creating some purpose, meaning, or value in the difficult experience they are having. Therapists might point out that it is essentially making lemonade from lemons.

Improving the Moment with *prayer* is very helpful for some clients. This means of improving the moment involves opening one's heart to a greater wisdom, to one's own Wise Mind—or whatever prayer means to the client. The prayer might involve asking for the strength to bear one's pain.

Improving the Moment with *one thing in the moment* involves focusing attention on just the one thing that you are doing in the current moment. This is basically the practice of Mindfulness. Because life is made up of a series of moments, reminding yourself to stay in just the moment you are in can make it easier to bear the pain rather than focusing on how long the crisis has already lasted or projecting how long it will continue to last.

Improving the Moment with a *brief vacation* includes activities such as taking a blanket to the park and sitting on it for a few hours; giving yourself a day to turn off your phone (including your cell phone or personal digital assistant) and letting the answering machine take the calls; going to the movies for an afternoon; and so forth. It is important for the therapists to remind clients that, as always, they must take into account what will be effective for them. Some individuals practice taking a vacation too often during a crisis, essentially using it as an ongoing escape. This skill, therapists clarify, is meant more for those whose tendency is to stay with the crisis or conflict until it ends, refusing any break at all. For them, especially, taking a breather can be very effective.

Improving the Moment with *encouragement* includes saying things to oneself such as "I can stand this," "This won't last forever," "I will make it," and/or "I am doing the best I can." Any type of cheerleading or inner reassurance is a very effective way of Improving the Moment.

 DISCUSSION POINT: *"What thoughts, comments, or reactions do you have to the Improving the Moment skill?"*

Therapists might use the following exercise to help clients experientially practice a Crisis Survival skill, modifying it as needed.

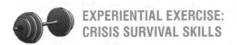 **EXPERIENTIAL EXERCISE: CRISIS SURVIVAL SKILLS**

"Get comfortable in your chair, your feet on the floor, your posture erect, and choose a place for your eyes to focus. Breathe several deep breaths from your diaphragm. Bring to mind a crisis of some sort—either one you are currently experiencing, one you have experienced in the past, or one you can imagine occurring in the future. Then imagine using one of the Crisis Survival skills. Perhaps you'd choose a Distraction skill, something to temporarily reduce your contact with the overwhelming situation. Perhaps an activity, contributing, or doing something that brings up an opposite emotion? Or imagine Self-Soothing being compassionate with yourself and doing something that pleases one of your senses. Or perhaps Improve the Moment you are in by using imagery or finding meaning in the situation. Remember, these skills won't solve the crisis, but they are ways to shore up oneself in order to bear pain more effectively."

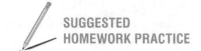

As with the other Distress Tolerance skills, it may be helpful for clients to track how effective each different Crisis Survival skill is so that eventually they will have an idea of which ones tend to be most helpful. Clients can keep notes of which categories of skills were used (e.g., Distracting, Self-Soothing, Improving the Moment), which specific skill was tried (e.g., taking a bubble bath as a way of Self Soothing with touch), and the distress experienced before (from 0–100) and after (from 0–100) a particular skill was used.

Therapists instruct clients to practice trying at least three different Crisis Survival skills each day over the following week or until the next session in order to become familiar with all of them.

Thinking of Pros and Cons

This Crisis Survival skill gives clients a chance to think, in a very deliberate way, of the pros and cons of tolerating their distress and the pros and cons of not tolerating it. It can be very helpful for surviving a crisis.

In thinking of the pros of tolerating the distress without engaging in a potentially self-destructive behavior, clients might first bring their attention to the positive consequences of tolerating their distress. For example, clients might imagine how good they will feel if they don't act impulsively in this moment. They might focus on the light at the end of the tunnel or their long-term goals and how good it feels to make progress toward them instead of feeling as if they are taking steps backward.

In thinking of the negative consequences of tolerating the distress, clients might reflect on the very real advantages of times when they act impulsively to try to avoid the pain of the current moment. Using food can really work to temporarily manage painful feelings and allow one to numb out or avoid them.

Clients should then direct their attention to thinking about the pros of not tolerating the distress. This may or may not be similar to the disadvantages of tolerating their distress without turning to food. The question to ask oneself is: What are the advantages of allowing myself to act impulsively and binge eat (and purge)?

Finally, clients should think about the disadvantages of not tolerating their distress. What has acting impulsively and binge eating (and purging) cost the clients in the past? What would it cost currently—or in the near future—in terms of their self-confidence, mood, relationships, physical well-being—their overall quality of life?

Therapists might use the following exercise to give clients the experience of practicing the skill of Thinking of Pros and Cons, modifying as needed.

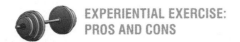

EXPERIENTIAL EXERCISE:
PROS AND CONS

"Take a piece of paper and pen. Take a moment to think about and write down the pros of tolerating, during a crisis, the distress you'd be experiencing. What are the benefits of acknowledging the reality of the pain and truly trying to survive the experience without making it worse? Then, what are the disadvantages of tolerating those emotions and not turning to solutions that will offer short-term relief? After considering those, write down the advantages of not tolerating the painful emotions and allowing yourself to impulsively turn to food or engage in another problematic behavior. Finally, identify and write down the disadvantages of not tolerating the pain, bringing to mind your experience over time, as well as its implications for the present and your future."

DISCUSSION POINT: *"What are you aware of by having filled this out? How do you want to respond next time you are facing a crisis?"*

TROUBLESHOOTING DIFFICULTIES
IN TEACHING CRISIS SURVIVAL SKILLS

- *Example 1*: "I don't understand when I should be using the Crisis Survival skills versus when I should be using Emotion Regulation or Mindfulness skills."
- *Potential therapist reply*: "The decision about when to use each skill is a Wise Mind type of decision. I'm not suggesting that you should always distract yourself, for example, or use one of the other Crisis Survival skills when dealing with your emotions. There are definitely times when you need to be acting based on your emotions. But at the times when you feel so overwhelmed that you cannot access your Wise Mind and you experience a strong urge to binge [and purge]—that is, you are in Emotion Mind—the Crisis Survival skills give you a way to just survive that moment without turning to behaviors that will not only not help you to respond effectively but will actually make matters worse. Binge eating [and purging] or pulling the covers over your head are ineffective responses because they compound the problem, leaving you faced with both the crisis and the negative consequences of binge eating [and purging]."
- *Example 2*: "I'm confused about the difference between distracting with opposite emotions and Acting Opposite [from the Emotion Regulation module]."
- *Potential therapist reply:* "That's an important question! The Distress Tolerance skill of distracting with an opposite emotion really focuses on getting a quick result to help you manage yourself through a crisis. It allows you to take a break. When you are using Acting Opposite as an Emotion Regulation skill, you are making a long-term change to address an emotion that isn't working for you. Temporarily, acting opposite of emotions you wish to change can cause increased distress—such as when you approach something, such as getting on an airplane, that you fear. But over time, the emotion will diminish if you continue to act opposite. The anxiety will decrease, for example, if a person continues to approach airplanes instead of avoiding them."

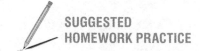

SUGGESTED
HOMEWORK PRACTICE

Therapists instruct clients to review, during the week, the Thinking of Pros and Cons that they wrote during the session. As clients face crises, be they big or small, and notice urges to turn to food, they should work through on paper additional pros and cons (e.g., pros of tolerating the distress, cons of tolerating the distress, pros of not tolerating the distress, cons of not tolerating the distress). Rating their distress (on a scale of 0–100) before and after practicing the skill will help clients evaluate its effectiveness for them.

List of Distress Tolerance Skills to Be Taught

- Observing Your Breath

- Half-Smiling

- Accepting Reality Awareness

- Radical Acceptance (Turning the Mind, Willingness versus Willfulness)

- Burning Your Bridges

- Crisis Survival skills (Distracting, Improving the Moment, Self-Soothing, Thinking of Pros and Cons)

Burning Your Bridges

Burning Your Bridges is accepting at a very deep level that you are never going to binge and/ or purge again. It is burning the "binge eating (and purging) bridge," the bridge that you've traveled across to allow yourself to engage in these behaviors. Burning that bridge means that binge eating (and purging) will no longer be an option, that you are making an active choice that this method will no longer be your way to "solve" your problems or cope with difficult situations when your emotions seem overwhelming. It is a radical concept because you are accepting that, *regardless* of your experience, the behavior of turning to binge eating (and purging) will not exist as an option. You are making a decision from deep within that there are other ways that you can regulate your emotions and that you must instead turn to them.

Burning Your Bridges can be paralleled with the experience of smokers who stop "cold turkey." It is that type of radically accepting one's experience. It is accepting and acknowledging that you are going to have painful and distressing experiences and emotions and that you will deal with them without the option of binge eating (and purging). It may also mean that you act to cut off all options that tend to lead you to binge eat and/or purge (apparently irrelevant behaviors, etc.). Depending on your particular circumstances, for example, it may mean disposing of the foods on which you binge.

Instructions: Describe what Burning Your Bridges means to you. Do you have a picture of a burning bridge? Are there steps you would want to take now to cut off the options? Use the remainder of this sheet, including the back, if you need extra space.

CHAPTER 7

Final Sessions

Review and Relapse Prevention

The final sessions of treatment are devoted to addressing several important issues. These include:

- Renewing clients' commitment to abstinence and using the skills instead of binge eating (and purging).
- Processing feelings associated with the treatment coming to an end.
- Reviewing the skills in order to emphasize their application and to underscore that practice is a lifelong endeavor.
- Discussing strategies for preventing posttreatment relapse.

There is much to cover, and therapists will need to be sensitive both to the needs of their particular group or individual client and to the importance of allowing adequate time to discuss the material.

RENEWING COMMITMENT TO ABSTINENCE AND USING THE SKILLS

As treatment nears to a close, it is vitally important that clients renew their commitment to abstinence from problematic eating behaviors and their commitment to using skillful means. The aim is to strengthen clients' resolve regarding the cessation of their binge eating (and purging) and the adoption of the skills in place of problem eating behaviors. With this in mind, therapists ask clients to recall the commitment they made at the start of treatment. How has this commitment influenced their behavior, thoughts, and experience? Allow a few clients to comment. Next, therapists might summarize their own perspectives along the following lines:

"Each of you had the courage to undertake this treatment and make a commitment to yourself to work toward cultivating a happier, more satisfying life, one in which you feel much better about yourself, more vital, more confident. You promised yourself that you would honor yourself by directly experiencing your life instead of using food to blunt or escape difficulties. Understandably, at times you may feel a sense of deprivation or loss when consciously deciding to relinquish the familiar habit of binge eating [and purging] to cope. Although these behaviors have some short-term 'upsides,' our discussions at the beginning of treatment led to the heartfelt insight and convincing conclusion that continuing to binge eat [and purge] was not compatible with living up to your fullest potential. You've learned that *not* acting on the urge to binge [and purge] is a great freedom and have felt empowered by your choice to turn to skills. You have become less driven by and reactive to your emotions and are instead developing a mindful awareness of what is taking place inside of you and responding with skillful means."

At this point, therapists might check with clients regarding any further comments. Next, it is vital that clients renew their commitment to abstinence. Therapists might say:

"Your commitment to abstinence from binge eating [and purging] is a critical foundation on which you are building a happier life. That foundation must be solid—the firm commitment that it is *not* an option to use food to cope with life's stresses. With that commitment firmly established, you are free to experiment with, explore, and apply the myriad adaptive skills you've learned in this treatment. Remind yourself of the increased flexibility that comes from living a life in which your behavior is not mood dependent, in which you have the freedom to *not* use food and to practice skillful means instead."

Offer clients the choice to express their recommitment out loud or silently to themselves. Suggest that clients reconnect with their commitment at least weekly, perhaps daily, once treatment ends.

TREATMENT TERMINATION

It is normal and to be expected that both clients and therapists will have many different thoughts and feelings about treatment coming to an end. It is important to acknowledge this to clients and to allow time for discussion. Underscore that the old habit of avoiding feelings is no longer an option. Termination provides an opportunity to experience and express feelings, using the skills accordingly. Therapists might begin the discussion along the following lines: "It is normal to feel some concern about the fact that therapy will be ending soon. Perhaps you are feeling anxious or sad. Or at times feeling a sense of pleasure that it will be over because you've gotten what you needed and feel ready to continue making progress on your own. Or perhaps there are other emotions you are experiencing ... ?"

Clients may express a sense of loss, which therapists can validate with something such as: "Of course! This is a group in which you've been supported and have been able to support others. Practice letting yourself maintain awareness of that experience without judging it."

Clients may experience anxiety as well. Highlight the importance of allowing awareness of such feelings: "Your fears are not something to talk yourself out of. If being in this group has helped you, it's understandable that you may be frightened about how you will maintain your commitment to your abstinence from binge eating [and purging] once treatment ends."

The key point is for clients to use the opportunity near the end of treatment to practice experiencing whatever emotions are coming up without turning to food. Unlike at other times in their lives, when they may have turned to food or other means to numb themselves to emotions with which they lacked skillful means of coping, clients no longer have to miss the chance to emotionally experience events in their lives—including the upcoming termination. Help clients to be as specific as possible about their feelings, pointing out that vague descriptions, such as "I'm feeling upset," may actually cover up more in-depth understanding. At this point in treatment clients can recognize times at which they are speaking to themselves in ways to avoid being close to their deeper emotional experiences.

 DISCUSSION POINT: *"What emotions are you aware of experiencing about the upcoming end of treatment?"*

REVIEW OF SKILLS

Explain that the purpose of the review is to strengthen skill acquisition, and underscore that if the skills are to be of benefit, practice is an ongoing, lifelong commitment. Emphasize that the skills are always an available option for clients to use if they turn their Wise Minds to them. It is particularly relevant to fortify practice of the skills, as more feelings regarding termination will likely surface after treatment ends.

Mindfulness Module

Begin the review of Mindfulness by emphasizing how the Mindfulness skills truly serve as the foundation for the rest of the skills clients were taught. This is why they are considered the core skills. The "What" and the "How" skills are the keys, the tools to accessing Wise Mind, and are cultivated on a daily basis. Initiate a brief discussion about the three states of mind: Reasonable Mind, Emotion Mind, and Wise Mind. For example, are clients able to identify what state of mind they are in? How do they use this information to direct their coping efforts? Have clients engaged in a regular practice of accessing their Wise Minds? If so, "What" do they do to find this state of mind? How does finding Wise Mind help clients realize their goals?

Briefly review the "What" skills, asking clients to describe each "What" skill in their own words. If needed, offer a few general points such as: *"Observe* involves stepping back from your experience, noticing without getting caught up in or clinging to that experience—allowing your experience to come and go. *Describe* involves putting words on experiences. It involves labeling a thought as a thought or putting a name to feelings." Remind clients of the tendency we all have to believe that because a thought enters one's mind, it *must* be true. However, obviously, this is not the case. By describing to oneself and labeling a thought as a thought, for instance, one is better able to have an objective stance toward one's experience. With Participate, clients are practicing being fully in the moment.

Review the "How" skills in a similar fashion, asking clients to describe each as if they were teaching it to a friend. If needed, therapists can add to the discussion with reminders such as:

> *"Nonjudgmentally* means ungluing opinions from facts, acknowledging but not judging, and looking at what has occurred—what *is. One-Mindfully* involves practicing patience in the moment. It is patiently bringing one's full attention to the present moment and keeping the mind from going off in multiple directions or becoming distracted. One-Mindfully is accepting the present, one moment at a time, while letting go of competing distractions. *Effectively* is focusing on what works. It is doing what needs to be done in each situation."

Remind clients that Effectively is not about what is fair or what is right or wrong. When being Effective, one's focus is on playing by the rules, keeping one's eye on one's objectives. Acknowledge that it may not be fair that clients have urges to binge (and purge) and others do not. Being Effective means playing with the cards one was dealt and not cutting off one's nose to spite one's face. Other potential questions for discussion might include:

- "'How' do you get to your Wise Mind?"
- "'How' do you focus your attention instead of remaining mindless and in the grip of Emotion Mind?"
- "'How' do you Observe, Describe, and Participate?"

The Mindfulness "What" and "How" skills underlie Mindful Eating, Urge Surfing, and Alternate Rebellion. *Mindful Eating* is eating with full awareness and attention and without self-consciousness or judgment. *Urge Surfing* entails the nonattached observing of urges to binge (and purge), riding the urge out without trying to block, stop, or fight it. *Alternate Rebellion* includes being effective by finding alternate means to rebel that do not involve binge eating. One uses rebelliousness in ways that do not backfire and result in greater difficulties. Encourage clients to describe their use of these skills, including times they have had trouble with them and times they have been able to use them to steer clear of binge eating (and purging).

Emotion Regulation Module

Enumerate each of the goals of the Emotion Regulation module, asking clients to reflect on one key idea that was important or meaningful to them for each of the following: (1) identify your emotions; (2) explore the function of your emotions; (3) reduce your vulnerability to Emotion Mind; (4) increase your positive emotions; (5) decrease your suffering by using Mindfulness to let go of distressing emotions; and (6) use Acting Opposite to emotion behaviors to change your emotional experience.

Include a review and discussion of the following ideas and skills: Observing and Describing one's emotions, experiencing one's emotions as a wave, and remembering that one is not one's emotion. The idea is to honor all one's experiences, not judging oneself or one's emotions, to reduce emotional suffering. Underscore that *Acting Opposite to the Current Emotion* can be a powerful way to change or reduce the intensity of an emotion that is interfering with the quality of clients' lives. For example, if clients feel down or depressed, they may avoid social engagement, potentially prolonging their negative moods. Acting Opposite to the Current Emotion would involve approaching the situation and opening the possibility of a different, positive experience. Acknowledge that this skill does not offer a "quick fix"; its benefits derive from repeated practice.

A sampling of questions to ask as part of the overall discussion include:

- "Which Emotion Regulation skills are your 'strongest'—the ones you feel most confident about being able to access?"
- "Which Emotion Regulation skills need more of your focus and practice? For example, is it easy to identify the action urge associated with an emotion but hard to clarify the interpretations you're using?"
- "What are the functions of emotions?"
- "How do binge eating [and purging] and other problematic eating behaviors interfere with the function of emotions? For example, how would binge eating when angry interfere with communication, organizing action, and self-validating?"
- "What have been your observations regarding the idea that fighting your experience tends to increase suffering?"
- "What has been your experience with Acting Opposite to the current Emotion?"
- "Think about the strongest emotion you experienced this past week. What were your body sensations, your action urges? Could you have changed your interpretation? Could you have changed your physical sensations?"
- "What has been your experience with reducing your vulnerability to Emotion Mind? What would be your current goals?"
- "What kinds of positive events have you been adding to your life?"
- "Have you been working to avoid avoiding?"
- "What has been your progress on your long-term goals (e.g., attending to relationships)?"

Distress Tolerance Module

Begin the review of this module by reminding clients of the idea underlying these skills—that pain is an inevitable part of life. The Distress Tolerance skills are aimed at helping clients endure distressing or uncomfortable situations without making the moment worse, such as through binge eating (and purging).

Distinguish between the two types of Distress Tolerance skills: Acceptance skills (e.g., Radical Acceptance, Observing Your Breath, Half-Smiling, and Awareness Exercises) and Crisis Survival skills (e.g., Distracting, Self-Soothing, Improving the Moment, and Thinking of Pros and Cons). Remind clients that turning to the Crisis Survival skills is not intended to solve the problem nor necessarily make it go away, but to help clients survive the crisis without making things worse.

Recall for clients that a crisis does not have to be huge in order for them to use their Crisis Survival skills. They can turn to them any time they have an urge to binge (and purge), eat mindlessly, or find themselves facing cravings.

Emphasize that Acceptance is not about passivity. Indeed, Acceptance may involve facing and acknowledging that change must take place.

In reviewing the Distress Tolerance module, therapists may wish to ask:

- "How would you describe in your own words why you need to learn Distress Tolerance skills? What are they good for? What is their rationale?"
- "How has learning the Distress Tolerance skills improved your ability to regulate strong emotional states?"
- "How have the Distress Tolerance skills replaced impulsive Emotion Mind behaviors such as bingeing [and purging]?"
- "What are the major categories of Crisis Survival skills? Which have you tended to use? Which do you plan to try more in the future?"
- "What has been your experience with thinking in terms of the Pros and Cons of tolerating distress?"
- "How have you used the Acceptance exercises, such as Observing Your Breath?"
- "What has been your experience with Half-Smiling?"

COPING AHEAD[1]

After the review, therapists present Coping Ahead, the last new skill to be taught. This skill is particularly useful at this juncture, with treatment ending. As opposed to writing a chain analysis of a problem eating behavior, in which the idea is to examine the past to try to better understand what could have been done differently, Coping Ahead aims to move that analysis into the future.

As therapists clarify, this skill is one to turn to when clients are anxious about how they may respond in a particular situation. For example, if clients know they are vulnerable during social events with plentiful food, clients might practice Coping Ahead to help them manage more effectively during the actual event. This

---

[1] This skill was termed "Mental Simulation" in the original DBT for BED and BN manual and research.

might entail imagining themselves going to an upcoming party, anticipating in detail what it would be like to experience urges to binge (and purge), and imagining in detail their use of skills to adaptively cope with those urges.

The key to Coping Ahead is to be very specific. Practicing Coping Ahead for the preceding situation, clients might imagine asking themselves what their Wise Mind would say. In addition, they might practice Radical Acceptance—rehearsing moving through the steps of Turning the Mind. They might also imagine identifying their emotions (e.g., anxiety, sadness) and examining their function. This might be followed by mentally simulating and practicing the skill of Burning Your Bridges to binge eating (and purging). Coping Ahead could also involve clients observing and developing new perspectives on the situation and on their responses.

Coping Ahead involves rehearsing in detail what clients would actually say to themselves and what they would actually do. By practicing Coping Ahead, clients may receive powerful reassurance that that they will be able to effectively use their skills to cope with difficult situations and that their emotional states do shift and pass. Emphasize that when clients mentally simulate turning to skills and surviving difficult situations, they are more likely to know what to do when actually facing these circumstances.

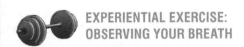 **EXPERIENTIAL EXERCISE: OBSERVING YOUR BREATH**

"Get into a comfortable position with your feet on the floor, head and spine straight, and breathe in and out from your diaphragm. Choose a spot on which to focus your eyes. Allow your mind to imagine a future situation in which you are likely to experience urges to binge [and purge], eat mindlessly, or engage in other problematic eating behaviors. This may be an actual upcoming situation or one that, based on your past experience, you can anticipate being difficult—such as a holiday celebration at which you typically overeat. Practice Coping Ahead by seeing yourself in detail experiencing the situation. Picture what you are doing, saying, and feeling. Mentally simulate turning to the skills to cope effectively with the situation. For example, imagine practicing Observing Your Breath as you find out what your available food choices are. Imagine seeking guidance from your Wise Mind. Really see yourself in detail practicing turning to the skills. As you do, observe whether any obstacles come up. If so, mentally simulate coping with those obstacles. For example, if you imagine that you might begin to overeat and experience the urge to capitulate and binge [and purge], mentally simulate Turning Your Mind toward the path of Willingness. Cope Ahead by remembering the skill of dialectical abstinence, radically accepting what you have done as you recommit to abstinence from this moment forward. Imagine identifying your emotions and thinking about their function. See yourself gaining a new perspective, handling the situation effectively, and being nonjudgmental with yourself. When you are ready, take several deep breaths and end the exercise."

 DISCUSSION POINT: *"What was your experience of Coping Ahead? Can you think of other future situations in which you might turn to this skill?"*

If time permits, the following general questions may be helpful as part of a final review:

- "What skills have you found most useful?"
- "Are there some that are particularly useful for certain instances, and others for different circumstances?"
- "Which skills did you find it difficult to practice or that need more practice?"
- "What interferes with your practice of those skills?"
- "Specifically, how have you used skills to replace binge eating [and purging], mindless eating, and other problematic eating behaviors?"

Planning for the Future

Distribute the Planning for the Future Homework Sheet (Appendix 7.1). Its goal is to help clients think specifically about strategies for maintaining treatment gains and for continuing to make further progress after treatment ends. In our research protocols, this handout is distributed in the second-to-last session to allow clients time to reflect, make plans, and discuss their plans during the final session.

Therapists might say:

"Here is a Planning for the Future sheet. We ask you to seriously consider the issues represented on it. Our next session is our last. During the second half of the session, each of you will have the opportunity to share parts of your Planning for the Future homework sheet. The handout asks you to describe your specific plans for continuing to practice the skills taught in the program. For example, you may decide to continue to keep the diary card as a record of your skills practice and set a goal to practice at least one skill each day. You might identify the five skills that you practiced the least and the five skills you found the most helpful and develop a plan to practice these each day.

"The second activity on this sheet involves identifying how you will deal with specific emotions in the future that previously set off problem eating for you. For example, have you often reacted to anger or anxiety by binge eating [and purging]? The purpose of having a plan is to be able to implement it to prevent any problem eating behaviors. We know that with the treatment program ending, the most important things for you will be to continue with your skillful behaviors and healthy eating and to maintain your abstinence from problem eating behaviors. As part of this exercise, you may also want to focus on remembering your typical dysfunctional links, the ones you've had to work through in the past. Was it the thought 'I deserve food' or 'It doesn't matter' or 'Food will help me feel better'? Which skills were most useful for dealing with these links? The third activity on the sheet is to write about what you need to do next to continue building a rewarding, satisfying way of life."

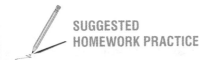

**SUGGESTED
HOMEWORK PRACTICE**

Therapists instruct clients to complete the Planning for the Future Homework Sheet (Appendix 7.1) and be prepared to discuss it at the next session.

FINAL SESSION

Therapists may wish to structure the final session similarly to that followed in our research studies. The first half of this last session, like preceding sessions, is devoted to reviewing each client's report of his or her skills practice and chain analyses of any problem eating behaviors.

After the break, clients are given the opportunity to provide feedback about their experience in treatment. This is followed by a review of each client's plan for the future. Good-byes are then said.

Feedback

Therapists may wish to use and/or adapt the following questions, introducing them by explaining: "Because we are continually developing this treatment program and hope to further improve, we would like to spend a few minutes finding out about your opinions and experiences."

- "How did this treatment program go for you?"
- "In what ways did the treatment help, and how did it fail to help you?"
- "Did you find input from other group members helpful?"
- "What has been important for you about the group?"
- "Would you have preferred to receive treatment on a one-to-one basis through individual treatment? [Or for those receiving individual treatment] Would you have preferred to receive treatment in a group therapy format?"
- "In your opinion, were there too little, too many, or just the right number of skills taught?"
- "Did you find the in-session practice exercises, such as the Mindful Eating exercise and Half-Smiling, to be helpful to you?"
- "How did the homework review portion work for you?"
- "What were your favorite skills?"
- "How did this treatment help in other areas of your life?"
- "Do you have any ideas on issues that we haven't yet discussed that would help improve the treatment program?"

Planning for the Future

Clients share their responses to the Planning for the Future homework sheet with the group.

Good-byes

Therapists may wish to say good-bye to the group by expressing admiration for clients' hard work and appreciation for their sharing and participation. This may be stated generally or with specific reference to each client. Communicate belief and confidence in the clients' abilities to continue to build a high quality of life for themselves, one that is free of problem eating behaviors.

In our experience, group members often take the initiative to give parting gifts to one another (e.g., a piece of heavy parchment paper with inspiring quotes, a CD with songs that group members would likely find moving and meaningful). (Note: Chapter 9, Future Directions, includes a discussion of handling the issue of relapse.)

Planning for the Future Homework Sheet

1. Write about specific plans you can put into place to help you continue to practice the skills that have helped you during this program.

2. Think of circumstances and emotions that previously tended to set off binge eating. For example, identify your typical prompting events, typical vulnerabilities, and typical dysfunctional links. Write about at least one of each and outline your plans for the skills you would use in each circumstance to deal with the typical emotions that are generated. In other words, how will you prevent a binge or other problem eating behavior? Please use the back of this page as needed.

Typical Prompting Events (e.g., dinner party, argument)

Typical vulnerabilities (e.g., overtiredness, alcohol)

Typical dysfunctional links (e.g., "What the heck," "I deserve this," "I can't stand this without eating," "I know the skills are there but I don't want to use them.")

3. Write about what you need to do next to continue building a satisfying and rewarding quality of life for yourself.

CHAPTER 8

Illustrative Case Examples

This chapter describes the application of DBT for BED and BN with two case examples. The aim of these examples is to illustrate a typical course of therapy and to offer guidance regarding issues likely to present the therapist with challenges. The first case example involves a client with BN whose treatment was delivered in an individual format (twenty 50- to 60-minute sessions). The second case example includes clients with BED who were treated via a group format (twenty 2-hour sessions).

Each treatment description includes the following:

- Pretreatment session
- Orientation to DBT (Sessions 1–2)
- Core Mindfulness module (Sessions 3–5)
- Emotion Regulation module (Sessions 6–12)
- Distress Tolerance module (Sessions 13–18)
- Review of skills and planning for the future (Sessions 19–20)

All clients whose treatment we describe consented to treatment and to having their case material used in scholarly publications and for training purposes.

UTILIZING DBT IN AN INDIVIDUAL FORMAT FOR A CLIENT WITH BN

Clinical Presentation

Sarah was a 36-year-old Caucasian woman who met criteria for BN according to the text revision of the fourth edition of the *Diagnostic and Statistical Manual of Mental Disorders* (DSM-IV-TR; American Psychiatric Association, 2000) and who was treated by one of us (D. L. S.).[1] Sarah lived with her husband and their two

---

[1]A version of this case was first published in Safer et al. (2001a).

daughters, ages 7 and 5 years. She worked part time as a shop assistant, and her husband worked full time as an engineer.

The Eating Disorder Examination (EDE; Fairburn & Cooper, 1993), a standardized interview for the assessment of eating-disorder diagnoses, was administered at baseline. According to the EDE classification, Sarah reported 13 "objective" (i.e., eating an unusually large amount of food while experiencing a loss of control) binge-eating episodes, 12 "subjective" (i.e., experiencing a loss of control while eating an amount of food that would not generally be regarded as excessive) binge-eating episodes, and 21 purging episodes over the preceding 28 days.

Sarah described being raised in a large family and recalled her mother as emotionally distant, seeming always preoccupied with caring for Sarah's multiple siblings and starting another new diet. She remembered feeling often that she had not been "heard" in her family. Sarah first began to diet in elementary school, portraying herself as slightly overweight and wanting to be thinner, "more like the other girls." Her binge eating and purging began when she was 23 years old. At that time she had just started working. Being away from home and away from her support network from college, she found herself feeling very lonely during the evenings. The course of her BN over the next 13 years waxed and waned but had steadily become more severe. At the time she came to treatment she weighed 109 pounds and was 5 feet 2 inches tall (BMI = 20 kg/m^2). She reported her lowest weight as an adult as 109 pounds and her highest weight as 125 pounds.

Sarah reported that her binge eating and purging worsened coinciding with a series of depressive symptoms occurring in the 4–6 months following the birth of her first child. During this period, 7 years prior to beginning the current treatment program, she was also physically disabled due to a shoulder injury. She sought counseling for 2 years. She found counseling helpful for her depressive symptoms, though with little effect on her bulimic symptoms. She had never received psychotropic medications. At the time Sarah sought treatment in our study, she did not meet clinical criteria for major depression nor for any other Axis I or II disorders, including current or past problems with alcohol or other substance abuse or dependence.

Although clients with BED and BN entering our treatment studies often present with a variety of comorbid conditions (see Table I.1), Sarah's case is presented to maintain primary focus on illustrating the typical delivery of DBT as adapted for BN. Her treatment consisted of 20 weekly 50- to 60-minute sessions of individual psychotherapy. The initial 20 minutes of each session involved a review of the homework/skills taught in the previous session, and approximately 30 minutes involved didactic teaching of new skills (see Chapters 3–7, this volume).

Orientation to DBT: Pretreatment Interview and Sessions 1–2

Pretreatment Interview

The pretreatment session (see Chapter 3) is an opportunity to build a collaborative relationship, to conduct some assessment of the presenting problem, to review the affect regulation model of binge eating–purging, and to elicit the details of a recent binge–purge episode. Additionally, the goals and targets of treatment are reviewed, followed by discussion of the therapist's and client's treatment agreements.

After a brief introduction and welcome to therapy, Sarah was asked about why she was seeking treatment at this point in time:

> "My bulimia is the worst it has ever been in my life. I'm worried about the effects of my behavior on my daughters' chances of developing eating disorders. This is not the role model I want to be. My bulimia is also making me ashamed of myself as a person and is affecting my marriage. I don't feel I can really talk with him about what I'm doing."

Sarah's treatment history was reviewed, and it was established that this was the first time she had sought treatment specifically for her eating disorder. As noted, she had previously sought counseling for her depressed mood, and at that time her eating behaviors were rarely if ever discussed. She was pleased that her prior treatment helped to relieve her depressed mood but was disappointed that it did not offer help for her eating-disorder symptoms.

Sarah was then introduced to the model of emotion dysregulation and was shown the form in Appendix 3.1 (Chapter 3). This model, as was explained, assumes an association between dysregulated emotions and dysfunctional eating-disordered behaviors. Sarah was asked to describe a recent binge–purge episode to determine the fit of the model for her problematic eating patterns. Sarah detailed an episode that had occurred the night before, and the therapist asked, "What do you think set it off?"[2]

SARAH: I was really stressed, tired from working in the morning and then taking care of the girls in the afternoon. I started thinking about binge eating when I was supervising my older daughter's homework. With school starting and my husband traveling so much, I feel really pulled in many directions—all I could start to think about was getting some time for myself and binge eating.

THERAPIST: So what I'm hearing is—it was a difficult day, work and the children were completely draining, and to top it off, your husband was gone. I'm guessing that you were feeling frustrated at how much was expected of you by your family and job, and maybe you were feeling lonely and unsupported by your husband, not having him there to share these burdens. According to our model, these emotions of frustration and loneliness are uncomfortable, and you don't think that you can handle them, so you turn to binge eating and purging, which in our model is the overlearned maladaptive behavior. Does that sound like I got it right?

SARAH: Exactly.

THERAPIST: How did it feel after you binged and purged?

SARAH: I felt much calmer and centered. Well, at least initially.

THERAPIST: Your experience does seem to fit with our model, in which binge eating and purging work to help you numb out and avoid unpleasant feelings. This

---

[2]Modified, rather than exact, transcriptions of sessions are reported due to space limitations.

makes you feel better, as you said, at least initially. The reason you are here is that there are longer term consequences, such as your shame about being a poor role model for your daughters and feeling less close to your husband and burdened by this secret that makes you feel that you're not the person you want to be. Does that seem right?

SARAH: Yes—I've never heard it explained exactly like that. I always thought my binge eating made no sense but I can see that, in an odd way, it does.

THERAPIST: This treatment will teach you more effective ways to cope with your emotions.

SARAH: That sounds wonderful!

With Sarah's assertion that the model explained her binge eating and purging cycle well and her expressed motivation to learn more, the goals and treatment targets of DBT were outlined (Chapter 3, Appendix 3.2). Sarah endorsed the stated treatment goals and targets and agreed that stopping binge eating and purging was her most important goal. Additionally, she understood that attending to any behavior that interfered with her therapy would be important for the treatment to run smoothly.

The therapist outlined the modules to be taught, as well as the general structure of each weekly 50- to 60-minute session. The Individual Client and Therapist Treatment Agreements (Chapter 3, Appendices 3.4 and 3.5) were then reviewed. As Sarah had no questions about these,[3] she was asked to take them home to think about them further before bringing them back. If she felt comfortable, she could sign them. If not, the therapist would be happy to discuss them in more detail at that time.

Introductory Sessions (Sessions 1–2)

SESSION 1

The goals of the first session were: (1) to elicit a commitment to abstain from bingeing and purging; (2) to present the biosocial model; (3) to orient the client to the diary card and chain analysis; and (4) to review the client and treatment agreements.

The client's commitment to abstinence from binge eating and purging is critical to obtain at the outset; hence, when Sarah returned, she was asked to further describe the effects of binge eating and purging on her life and to outline her treatment goals. Sarah described feeling that her life was "in control in so many ways." She had daughters she loved, a good overall relationship with her husband, and a satisfying job. The bulimic behavior seemed the only aspect that was out of control. She also reported feeling that her eating disorder was a furtive secret she had been hiding from others, including her husband, for a long time. Although her bulimia had felt like her "best friend" when Sarah started engaging in it, over time it had become a highly distressing and lonely burden.

---

[3]Sarah did not bring up concerns about potential weight gain, although many clients with eating disorders do. Therapists can tell them that most bulimic clients do not experience much weight increase, if any ("usually not more than a couple of pounds"), after ceasing binge eating and purging.

The following exchange illustrates how the therapist encouraged Sarah's commitment to her goal of abstinence.

THERAPIST: From what you've told me, it really sounds like the bingeing and purging is having a significant negative impact on many important areas of your life. Does that feel true?

SARAH: Oh yes. Very true. It used to be such a comfort and would make me feel less stressed out. But now it seems to have a life of its own. I feel guilty and lonely, and it doesn't really help me with the stress, at least not for very long at all.

THERAPIST: I understand. It really does sound like it seriously interferes with the quality of life you want. However, despite the negatives, there are clearly some reasons why you continue doing it. Can we make a list of what some of the benefits of continuing might be?

SARAH: Well, there aren't too many. But I guess ... well ... when I get all stressed out and overwhelmed by trying to juggle the kids' homework, my job, trying to be both parents when my husband's job takes him out of town—that's when the bulimia can make me feel kind of more relaxed just after I've done it.

THERAPIST: I see. It helps, at least in the short run, to distract you from the stress and release some of the tension. Any other upsides?

SARAH: I get lonely when my husband's out of town, so it can be kind of a comfort.

THERAPIST: That's important—again. The bingeing and purging seems to serve to distract you from difficult feelings. And it's temporarily successful.

SARAH: I kind of get to have my cake and eat it, too, and not put on weight. That's also good.

THERAPIST: Hmm. I know you're here because you want to stop, but I have to say, there is a lot that works about the bulimia. Perhaps you should reconsider. Maybe there's a way to work out continuing to binge eat and purge and *also* develop a life really worth living. Do you think that's possible, rather than trying to eliminate the binge eating and purging?

SARAH: (*Is silent for a moment, then protests.*) I don't think you're getting it right. See, even if it makes me less stressed out just after I vomit, I still have to go back out there and somehow juggle everything. And because vomiting takes so much out of me, I'm so exhausted that I don't do as well as I could. Like I'm such a mess afterward I can't think straight. And even if it makes me less lonely when Dave is out of town, I'm married to Dave—and not to sticking my head down the toilet. And it's awful because I can't even bring myself to tell him about it—so having bulimia makes me even lonelier. He'd be so upset if he found out—not only because of how it is affecting my health but because he'd feel like I'd been cheating on him. We've shared everything in our relationship but this. And eating what I want and not putting on weight. Well, I hardly actually enjoy the food when I'm binge eating. And vomiting is gross. It makes your breath smell. Even if it's helping to control my weight I'm not sure I look good—the truth is I just look and feel worn out. No. Having bulimia and having the life I want to live—I just can't do both—I've tried and you can't do it.

THERAPIST: I can hear the defeat in your voice. That you've tried to have both the bulimia and a life that's meaningful for you, and it has not worked out. They're not compatible.

SARAH: They're not.

THERAPIST: Well, you've convinced me. OK—then that's it. From what you've said, there's no other way. You've got to stop the binge eating and vomiting and you've got to stop them now.

SARAH: Now?

THERAPIST: Yes—the last binge and vomit you had—we're going to christen them your last.

SARAH: Really? But I can't just stop it like that.

THERAPIST: Why not?! I don't see that you have much choice. You can't juggle all the things you do, have a completely honest relationship with your husband, deal with your job and the kids, and be the kind of mother you want to be—unless you stop the binge eating and vomiting. I'm convinced from what you've said that if you keep binge eating and vomiting, things will only get worse. Your only hope is to stop the binge eating and vomiting.

SARAH: Okay. Well, I do want to stop it, that is why I came. ...

THERAPIST: You don't sound so sure. Really consider what it means to give up the pros that the bingeing and purging temporarily offer. There may even be others that we haven't discussed. However, remember that the aim of this treatment is to teach you skills to manage all the stress and difficult emotions you describe. In the meantime, while you learn and practice the new skills, you'll need to draw on whatever skillful resources you already have but that may be rusty at this point.

SARAH: Well—I could try to stop.

THERAPIST: That's a great place to start. But we know from research and our experience that it takes more than trying to stop binge eating and purging. You need to make a genuine commitment—from the deepest part of yourself. A commitment from the part of you that wants to live up to your potential, be the kind of role model for your daughters that you respect, and have a healthier and more open relationship with your husband. Do you feel you can make that commitment?

SARAH: Yes, I can commit to stopping bingeing and purging. But I'm so afraid I won't be able to keep that commitment. What if I binge and purge after I leave?

THERAPIST: We're not asking you to predict the future. We're just asking that you make a commitment right here, right now, in this moment, to stop. After all, life is just a series of moments, and we have the opportunity to recommit from moment to moment.

SARAH: Well, OK. I can commit right now.

THERAPIST: That's a brave thing to do.

Following this, Sarah and the therapist reviewed the Individual Client and Therapist Treatment Agreements (Chapter 3, Appendices 3.4 and 3.5). Sarah was reminded of the structure of future sessions, with the first 20 minutes devoted to reviewing homework and the remaining 30 minutes devoted to learning new skills.

The therapist then introduced the chain analysis (Chapter 3) and explained that using this chain is a skillful behavior. Sarah was given instructions for completing the chain. This began by reviewing the path to mindful eating hierarchy (Chapter 3, Appendix 3.2), clarifying that the highest targets on the path (e.g., binge eating and purging) were to be written about before those lower on the list (e.g., apparently irrelevant behaviors). The role of the prompting event, or environmental trigger that precipitates the chain of problematic behaviors, was discussed, as well as vulnerability factors (e.g., lack of sleep, physical illness). The *links* of the behavioral chain, which include a client's *actions, body sensations, cognitions, events*, and *feelings*, were reviewed, and more skillful behaviors to replace the problem behaviors were identified. Sarah was directed to complete at least one chain analysis (Chapter 3, Appendix 3.8) prior to the next session with the help of the sample chain and guidelines (Chapter 3, Appendices 3.6 and 3.7).

Finally, Sarah was given a diary card and instructions for filling it out (Chapter 3, Appendices 3.9 and 3.10) and asked to record the frequency of targeted behaviors (e.g., binge eating and purging), to rate the presence and intensity of various emotional states, and to note which skills were practiced each day. She was told that at each session this would be reviewed, so it was important that she bring it weekly.

SESSION 2

This session's goals included reviewing the homework and teaching the new skills of dialectical abstinence and diaphragmatic breathing (see Chapter 3). The session began with a review of Sarah's diary card. Sarah had filled the card out for 4 of the previous 7 days. She said that she did not fill her card out for 3 days because she had binged and purged on those days and felt too ashamed to write about these behaviors. She also did not fill out a chain analysis.

The therapist explained that the incomplete homework was an example of therapy-interfering behavior and suggested that she and Sarah fill out a chain analysis together to better understand Sarah's not completing all of her homework.

THERAPIST: As we discussed last time, anything that stops you from participating in treatment is our number one priority. (*Brings out a blank chain analysis form.*) So, how was it that you didn't fill in Saturday, Sunday, and Monday of your diary card?

SARAH: I just couldn't. (*Looks down and becomes quiet.*)

THERAPIST: Tell me about what happened.

SARAH: The truth is that when I made the commitment not to binge I thought it would not happen ever again.

THERAPIST: It sounds like shame got in the way of you and the diary card.

SARAH: Well, yes—I guess.

THERAPIST: You'll be learning a new skill today that I think will really help you to cope with this shame without having to avoid your homework. Now, let's do a chain of your last binge.

The therapist and Sarah conducted a chain analysis of her previous binge and purge.

After reviewing homework, the therapist turned to teaching new skills. The therapist reassured Sarah that many clients find it difficult to cope with continued binge eating and purging despite their commitment to stop and explained that the skill of dialectical abstinence is specifically taught at this juncture to help clients understand, perhaps in a way they never have, the possibility of reinforcing their commitment to a goal even when they fail to reach that goal in the moment.

It was suggested that the skills, dialectical abstinence and diaphragmatic breathing, in addition to the diary card and chain analysis, were tools that Sarah could use to help her when she experienced urges to binge and purge during the following week.

Core Mindfulness Module: Sessions 3–5

In these sessions, Sarah was taught core mindfulness skills to increase her ability to be aware of and experience her feelings without reacting to them by engaging in emotion-driven eating behaviors (e.g., binge eating and purging). Specific skills taught included the "What" skills, the "How" skills, Mindful Eating, Urge Surfing, and Alternate Rebellion.

Vignette: Teaching Urge Surfing with a Malt Ball

THERAPIST: Take one of the malt balls, if you would. But don't eat it.

SARAH: I'm so scared!

THERAPIST: I know this is frightening. Although the urges feel overwhelming, what is freeing about learning to Urge Surf is learning that you can have an urge but not act on it.

SARAH: I'm with you now and am OK, but what will happen once I leave the session? I'll probably go out and binge!

THERAPIST: You're very worried, which is understandable. Take a few diaphragmatic breaths. What does your Wise Mind say about practicing this exercise?

SARAH: Well ... my Wise Mind thinks it makes sense. But I'm worried about what's going to happen after the end of the session.

THERAPIST: Let's do this exercise now, and we'll check in closer to the end of the session to see how you're doing. (*Proceeds with Urge Surfing experiential exercise.*)

Toward the end of the session, the therapist inquired: "Just checking in before we end today's session. Are you feeling any urges now to binge?"

SARAH: Yes! I'm a 6 out of 6 on my urges to binge scale!

THERAPIST: At this moment your urges are really strong. OK. What skills can you practice to manage these urges to binge?

SARAH: I guess I could sit outside in the waiting area and practice Urge Surfing and not leave the waiting room till my urges are reduced.

THERAPIST: That sounds good. Sometimes it takes longer than the time we have together in session for urges to decrease.

SARAH: My urges had decreased earlier but just went up when I realized the session was about to end.

THERAPIST: Anything that might interfere with this plan?

SARAH: Well—I might have to leave to pick up my kids before my urges go down.

THERAPIST: If that were to happen, what skill could you practice?

SARAH: Well, I could practice Mindfulness while I am at stoplights, Observing and Describing the steering wheel and how it feels in my hands.

THERAPIST: That sounds like a great solution. Do you think you can be committed to our plan—sitting in the waiting room till your urges go down, and then practicing Observe and Describe with the steering wheel at stoplights should you have to leave early?

SARAH: I'm committed to our plan.

Vignette: Teaching Alternate Rebellion

THERAPIST: I'm very excited to teach you this next skill because I think you'll find it particularly helpful at night, when you've described having lots of urges. It is called Alternate Rebellion. (*Explains the concept of alternate rebellion and then continues.*) How do you think binge eating and purging may be a form of rebellion for you?

SARAH: Oh, I'm not the rebel type!

THERAPIST: I hear you, but just go with me on this. I could be wrong, but I noticed you typically start having urges to binge at night when you're alone with the kids because Dave's still at work. The kids are making demands on you— they want dinner, they want help with their homework, they can't find their clothes for soccer practice tomorrow, and so on. I think anyone under the circumstances would feel just an itsy bitsy feeling of resentment, just a wee bit of feeling grumpy and annoyed, just even a little bit (*smiling*)?

SARAH: Well … maybe. I hate to think of myself being like that, but I think it's probably true. Sometimes I just want to run away from it all.

THERAPIST: How could you honor that very legitimate wish in a way that, unlike binge eating and purging, wouldn't harm you? Think of all the possibilities, even the wildest ones!

SARAH: I guess I could get some babysitting help. When I'm really stressed I could give up trying to push the homework till I felt better and instead watch a video with the kids.

THERAPIST: Great! Anything even more wild?

SARAH: I could have a juice spritzer with one of those paper umbrellas in it (*laughing*). I could read a celebrity magazine. Now that I think of it—it all sounds pretty good.

THERAPIST: These are excellent ideas for Alternate Rebellion! So what I'm understanding is that you turn to bingeing and purging to manage feeling stressed and maybe even the smallest bit (*smiling*) resentful. And in the short term it helps. But by practicing Alternate Rebellion, you are honoring your feelings and the urges to rebel and take care of yourself, but you do so without the longer term guilt and shame that your bingeing and purging is causing.

Emotion Regulation Module: Sessions 6–12

By the sixth session, Sarah reported having stopped engaging in large binges and compensatory purges. She still struggled, however, with smaller binges (i.e., subjective binges). The goals of this next module are to teach the client how to identify and label her or his emotions, understand the function of her or his emotions, reduce her or his vulnerability to intense emotions, increase the number of positive emotional events, increase mindfulness of emotions, and learn to change her or his emotional experience when possible.

In discussing the model of emotions (Chapter 5, Appendix 5.2), Sarah said that she did not think that emotions sometimes really played a role in her urge to vomit—it was more the physical discomfort of having food in her stomach. Sarah's focus on physical rather than emotional sensations is typical of many bulimic clients.

SARAH: Like I was saying, I don't think any emotions are involved sometimes. I just feel physically uncomfortable—I can *feel* the bagel just sitting in my stomach, not moving! This model of emotions doesn't make sense when what's going on is purely physical.

THERAPIST: But in your voice I hear something more.

SARAH: It just feels gross and lumpy, and it makes my tummy stick out. But that's a physical thing.

THERAPIST: Hold on (*smiling*). I hear a judgment in the word "gross."

SARAH: Well, it just embarrasses me that my stomach is so poochy.

THERAPIST: Aha! Embarrassment is an emotion.

SARAH: But I'm not just embarrassed. It's really very uncomfortable.

THERAPIST: Let's look again at this model. Can you see how the event was eating the bagel and that, following this, the interpretation was "My stomach is gross"? This is associated with changes in your brain and body, and you find yourself focusing on those sensations and the interpretation again and again. All those are part of the embarrassment that you are describing, which starts to include shame. This is a great example of how emotions, such as embarrassment and shame, loving themselves, fire and refire again and again.

SARAH: Well, I guess that could be true. Some days, such as when I'm busy, I don't even notice what my stomach feels like when I've had a bagel.

In Session 8 the therapist discussed with Sarah the various functions of emotions. The therapist asked: "Based on what we've been talking about, how has binge eating and purging interfered with the natural function of your emotions?"

SARAH: Well, I don't know, really.

THERAPIST: One thing I have noticed is that you've mentioned that everyone around frequently comments on how "together" you are and how you seem to be able to do it all so effortlessly. Even my experience working with you is that it is hard for you to let me know that things are not as together as they seem.

SARAH: That is true—but people don't know the real me.

THERAPIST: It sounds as though you're on to something—that your binge eating and purging allow you to keep a happy face on so that people don't know the real you and the struggles that you have in juggling everything.

SARAH: I think that's true. And I don't want to use the binge eating and purging any more—the cost is too high.

In Session 9, as part of the discussion of vulnerability to Emotion Mind, the topic of balanced eating was brought up. One way that this adapted version of DBT differs from other treatments for eating disorders, such as CBT, is that it contains no behavioral focus on the pattern of eating. According to CBT's dietary restraint model, restriction of food leads to binge eating and purging. In DBT, hunger (or imbalanced food intake in general) is understood as increasing one's vulnerability to Emotion Mind but not as a prompting event per se.

THERAPIST: Does imbalanced eating make you more vulnerable to your Emotion Mind?

SARAH: I try to eat healthily.

THERAPIST: You do! One thing I've noticed from your recent chains is that you're likely to describe urges to binge while making dinner, especially if dinner is being prepared late.

SARAH: That's true. Evenings are a very busy time, with getting the girls fed, dinner made, and just dealing with the end of the day. If I'm too hungry on top of everything, I'm a lot more likely to feel overwhelmed and feel like bingeing.

THERAPIST: So, what could you do differently, based on your Wise Mind?

SARAH: Well, I guess not to ever get too hungry, especially not leaving dinner till really late.

Session 9 also involved discussion of Sarah's ratio of positive to negative experiences. The issue of hunger was brought up again. The focus was on emotions, with hunger (or food restriction) understood as a means of Emotion Regulation. For example, Sarah recognized that one of the ways she tried to generate a positive emotional experience, especially on very stressful days, was by staying hungry as long as she could because this felt "virtuous" and "good."

THERAPIST: Staying hungry appears to be a way of trying to regulate your emotions (*with teasing tone*). How could "staying hungry" not be on this pleasant events list? (*Waves handout back and forth.*)

SARAH: (*Laughs.*) I guess it's probably not there because it doesn't always work that well.

THERAPIST: In what way?

SARAH: Well, it makes me more crabby. I also notice I can't think very well because I feel so hungry.

THERAPIST: Do you think that eating as little as possible, just like purging, is an attempt to distance you from your emotional experiences of the day? From what I hear, I notice that you don't end up doing many pleasant activities during a day that are just for you. So instead of observing the emotions that you are experiencing over a day, your mind is focused on how little you have been eating.

SARAH: I wish it weren't true, but that makes sense.

In Session 11, the therapist and Sarah reviewed the myths about emotions.

THERAPIST: Which myth about emotions do you find most difficult to challenge?

SARAH: "Letting others know that I am feeling bad is weakness."

THERAPIST: (*with teasing tone*) Yes, asking your husband to unload the dryer maybe once a year to help you out a bit. That would be really weak!

SARAH: (*Laughs.*) Oh, asking Dave to unload the dryer once in a while wouldn't show him I'm weak. But I see what you're getting at. Maybe telling Dave about how stressed I am and how I need his help once in a while isn't such a sign of weakness. I like feeling like my needs are legitimate—it feels better than binge eating and purging to try to get rid of them.

Distress Tolerance Module: Sessions 13–18

During this third and final module, Sarah was taught Distress Tolerance skills (Acceptance skills and Crisis Survival skills) to help her tolerate painful emotions when distressing situations and circumstances took place that could not be changed in the moment. The Acceptance skills emphasize accepting one's current situation and emotional state from deep within. They include Observing Your Breath, Half-Smiling, using Awareness Exercises, and Radical Acceptance—which contains Turning the Mind and Willingness). The Crisis Survival skills involve the strategies of Distracting, Self-Soothing, Improving the Moment, and deliberate consideration of the Pros and Cons of either tolerating the distress or using maladaptive behaviors such as binge eating and purging.

In Session 16, the therapist presented the skill of Burning Your Bridges by leading Sarah in an experiential exercise. Sarah did not have difficulty deciding to burn her bridge to binge eating. She had ceased binge eating and purging for the preceding 10 weeks. Especially for those clients who may not have stopped by this point, the skill of Burning Your Bridges can be just what is needed to motivate a client to do so, making use of the fact that one more month of treatment remains (as per our research protocol of 20 sessions).

For example, consider another client, who was still struggling with binge eating and purging at this stage. She is asked whether she feels ready to burn her bridges to Binge Eating Island as a strategy to stop binge eating.

THERAPIST: I am thinking that this skill might really help you right now. What do you think about burning your bridges to stop binge eating and purging?

CLIENT: I'm scared. I'm still binge eating and purging every once in a while, which is a real improvement. It's hard to think of giving it up completely.

THERAPIST: I noticed how scared you are, too. But what I am thinking is that in order for you to gain confidence to deal with your fear without avoiding, we have to see what life is like without this behavior. I want to be with you when you do that—and we've got four sessions left to work on this together.

CLIENT: Well, the skills have worked when I have used them. But burning my bridges feels a little like jumping off a cliff.

THERAPIST: Can you tolerate that feeling and do it anyway?

CLIENT: I think I could. ... Oddly, I kind of feel excited. It seems like a second chance at committing to stopping binge eating and purging.

Continuing with the case description of Sarah, Session 17 involved teaching the Crisis Survival skills. Like many clients, Sarah expressed some apprehension when introduced to the set of Self-Soothing skills.

SARAH: I don't really like to see my body or touch it with lotions. It doesn't sound very soothing to me.

THERAPIST: Do you think you could give it a go just to make sure? Remember when using this skill to try to really throw yourself fully into it One-Mindfully. If your mind wanders to judgments about your body, for example, try to bring your mind back to experiencing the moment, such as focusing on the smell of the lotion or how it feels on your skin.

SARAH: OK. Maybe I'll surprise myself and enjoy it. And it makes sense that I need to learn how to find things other than food soothing!

Review of Skills and Planning for the Future: Sessions 19–20

In Sessions 19 and 20, the therapist and Sarah reviewed skills from the three previous sessions. In addition, plans were discussed to help Sarah prevent relapses once treatment ended. This involved having Sarah fill out a Planning for the Future Homework Sheet (Chapter 7, Appendix 7.1) to discuss during the following session.

In Session 20, when the therapist and Sarah reviewed her plan for the future, Sarah identified anger, hopelessness, and being ashamed as the emotions she found most difficult to tolerate and, therefore, most in need of a plan.

THERAPIST: What did you write down as specific plans for practicing the skills?

SARAH: I've decided to photocopy the diary card so I can have it near my bed to fill out every day. I think that would really help.

THERAPIST: Fantastic! Anything else?

SARAH: I've decided to take up yoga. I've always wanted to, and I think it would help me to keep practicing the Mindfulness skills.

THERAPIST: I agree! What about your plans for dealing with the specific emotions you mentioned?

SARAH: For when I'm angry, my plan is to turn to diaphragmatic breathing first, as that has always helped. Then I would access my Wise Mind to help me not to judge myself for how I feel. I also think Alternate Rebellion would help me to find ways to express my anger without hurting myself. For hopelessness, I plan to remind myself that I can Turn the Mind, I don't need to capitulate, and I can look at my diary card to remind me of all the skills I know now. And, finally, when I'm ashamed and feeling self-critical, I will use Radical Acceptance and a nonjudgmental stance. I may continue to feel these feelings, but I want to be aware of them. Also, from all the chains we did together, I think I've learned that not being too hungry is really important for me. So no matter what difficult emotion I'm experiencing, I would try to check out my vulnerabilities to my Emotion Mind and keep working on getting enough sleep and trying not to do it all.

Outcome of Treatment

Sarah's primary treatment target was to stop binge eating and purging. The information reported on the weekly diary cards indicated that after 5 weeks of treatment, Sarah had ceased bingeing and purging, and she continued to be free from objective bingeing and purging through the remainder of the 20 weeks. During the posttreatment interview, Sarah expressed appreciation for the treatment approach and stated, "This therapy taught me skills that I can use in difficult times. The skills help me to stop and reevaluate all situations [and to] deal more effectively with them." At the end of treatment Sarah had gained 4 pounds from her pretreatment weight. At 6-month follow-up, she reported two objective binges and two purges since ending treatment (an average of one binge-and-purge episode every 3 months). Sarah reflected positively on her experience over these months and explained that, rather than using food to help her manage her emotions, the therapy had taught her to identify her emotions and subsequently to utilize skills she had learned, such as diaphragmatic breathing, Wise Mind, and Radical Acceptance. Her weight was 114. However, she denied any feelings of dissatisfaction with her weight and reported instead that she felt healthy and fit. Her low weight of 109 was not worth the emotional costs of binge eating and purging.

UTILIZING DBT IN A GROUP FORMAT FOR CLIENTS WITH BED

Orientation to DBT: Pretreatment Interview and Sessions 1–2

Pretreatment Interview

The pretreatment interview, in which each prospective group member meets individually with one of the cotherapists, is similar to the pretreatment interview for the BN case described. The purpose of the interview was to orient the group member to treatment, to describe the model of affect regulation, to emphasize the goals and targets of treatment, and to review client and therapist agreements. In addition, the therapist should inquire about any prior experience in group therapy, go over guidelines for the group to run smoothly, and address any concerns about group treatment.

Commonly, very obese clients express the worry that they will be the heaviest clients in the group, as in the following vignette:

THERAPIST: Do you have any worries or concerns about being in the group that we haven't yet discussed?

CLIENT: Well, one thing I'm worried about is—will I be the heaviest one in the group?

THERAPIST: That's a really important question. Our groups include people who are a range of weights—from average to very overweight individuals. Although I cannot tell you for certain the weights of all the individuals in the group at this point, all of you will have something important in common. Everyone in this group struggles with binge eating.

CLIENT: But people who are thin wouldn't understand what it's like.

THERAPIST: It sounds like this feeling of not being understood could be one of the emotional experiences that leads to binge eating for you. Everyone in the group struggles with difficult emotions and a sense of defeat regarding how to cope without using food. So regardless of weight, the common factor binding the group together is the recognition that binge eating is causing great harm and the resolve to stop a behavior that only increases one's suffering in the long run. That's why we focus on getting the binge eating under control first and foremost.

Session 1

A primary goal of the first group session, as with the BN case presented, was to motivate clients to commit to binge abstinence. Additionally, the first session was designed to review the biosocial model, to discuss the client and treatment agreements, and to orient clients to the diary card and chain analysis form. When treatment is delivered in a group format, group dynamics can influence the process of obtaining a commitment to binge abstinence. The following excerpt from one of our group sessions illustrates a typical client with BED who was cautious about being able to commit to stop binge eating.

COTHERAPIST 1: What do you think about the pros and cons we've listed so far?

CLIENT 1: I'm living on the con side, there's no question about it. Because when I was younger and doing ten times as much and raising a family, I had more mental drive to make a change, and I could do it. I did a lot of things very successfully. Now, as much as I want this, I don't know if I can switch that on again.

COTHERAPIST 1: Sounds like you're afraid this will just be another task to add to your list, and you're not sure you have it in you to give the amount of effort it will take.

CLIENT 1: It does take a lot of energy, and it's like your engine needs a tune-up or something. You know, you just can't floor it. ... I've lived with this for so long, I'm finding that I am really struggling with making this commitment.

COTHERAPIST 1: It's understandable that as you look back on difficulties you had to contend with when you were younger and the amount of mental drive it required, you feel hesitant to tackle another issue. However, the treatment is designed to provide you with skills and tools that will eventually reduce the struggle and offer you some peace.

CLIENT 1: Back then I didn't have any skills. It was survival in a way. My motivation was that I was raising two children and wanted them to grow up well, have a happy home, be successful and so forth. ... I guess I had a payoff. But now those things are done!

COTHERAPIST 1: Sounds like when you put your mind to it, you can accomplish goals that you value. What would be the payoff now?

CLIENT 1: That's a good question. No one else is depending on me, it's a personal thing. I don't feel the drive right now that I used to feel.

COTHERAPIST 1: Any other thoughts, group?

CLIENT 2: Well, I think all the cons themselves are disgusting.

COTHERAPIST 2: So that's the payoff for you, to just get rid of the cons. (*To Client 1*) It appears you're fearful that there isn't something strong enough to compel you to change. Before, there were a lot of demands pressing on you and goals for your family that drove you to stop back then. Whereas now, maybe you are saying you've settled on a lower quality of life. You're not sure whether you have the inner "oomph" to do it—or "floor it" as you said. It is scary to think of trying to do this just for you. I mean it's certainly hard to embark on something like this.

CLIENT 1: Well, you know, that's a good point. Because it wasn't ever about me, at least not that I was aware of. It was always about something or someone else. And now that those something elses have been taken care of, we're back to the bare roots now. What I was hiding behind by using the binge eating, overworking, doing all those other things, I don't know, but now, the fundamental issue is still there.

COTHERAPIST 1: Perhaps the fundamental issue is allowing something of value for yourself, such as the skills we'll be teaching. Taking in something that benefits you in the long run and not approaching this from a pressured, demanding stance but from a more generous mind-set.

At this point the therapists opened up the discussion to include other group members' thoughts about making their commitment to group abstinence.

CLIENT 3: I feel the need to get back control. Every so often I feel as though I'm there but then I lose it. So I'm worried about being able to say I'm committed, because I've said that to myself before, but then I worry I won't stay with it.

COTHERAPIST 1: That's OK. What we're asking you is to just stay in this one moment. When you think of your goal or your intention, can you say at this moment, "Yes, I am committed at this moment to do everything I can to stop binge eating. That's why I'm here."

CLIENT 3: Yes.

COTHERAPIST 1: Great! (*Turns to next client.*)

CLIENT 2: I'm committed to trying my absolute best to stop binge eating because the consequences are so awful. But I know there will be times when I'll want the comfort of bingeing. To actually ask me to give that up is scary because no one really has. It's weird, to give something up that's such a part of you.

COTHERAPIST 2: There are amazing benefits to stopping, but there's no doubt it's scary to give up bingeing.

CLIENT 2: It's so numbing.

COTHERAPIST 2: Yes. As you sit here in this moment, can you say that you commit to stopping binge eating?

CLIENT 2: Yes.

COTHERAPIST 2: Great!

CLIENT 1: I have no idea how, but I'm willing to make the commitment!

COTHERAPIST 1: That's wonderful!

CLIENT 4: I feel like I'm totally committed, but I also stopped and had a very big lunch before I got here just because I felt I would need something.

COTHERAPIST 1: As you sit here in this moment, do you feel you can make the commitment?

CLIENT 4: Yes.

COTHERAPIST 1: OK, great.

Session 2

As discussed in Chapter 3, a particular challenge of the group format involves reviewing each client's homework in a timely manner. Following are ways to address the therapy-interfering behavior of clients who do not complete their homework for various reasons.

COTHERAPIST 1: What we'd like to do is have each of you—for about five to six minutes per person—take out your diary cards and tell us about your practice of skills this past week. Mary [Cotherapist 2] will keep track of time. This week that might include talking about renewing your commitment to stop binge eating or using the 3" × 5" card and really focusing on the negative consequences of binge eating. Then give us the highlights of the chain analysis you filled out, the key parts that you think are critical and that you'll need to change in order to stop binge eating. If you had any questions or problems filling this out, this is the time to ask. If you didn't complete the diary card or chain, we do ask that you fill those out and turn them in during the break. So, who's going to be the brave beginner and start out?

Example 1: "I had 'a week from hell.'"

CLIENT: I'm going to start off by using the excuse that this has been a week from hell—but it really has! I haven't done all of my homework, including not filling out any days on my diary card. This is very important, I realize, but I didn't get to it.

COTHERAPIST 1: Well, this is a good place to start, then. If you haven't completed your homework—whether because you didn't understand it or didn't get to it—that's going to interfere with your receiving the most benefit from treatment. As we talked about in the pretreatment orientation and again last week, that's the first thing we have to address, even before focusing on stopping binge eating. We've got to figure out what you think is getting in the way.

CLIENT: I didn't fill it out at all last week so I don't even know what exactly was going on.

COTHERAPIST 1: Let's look at just one instance of not filling out your diary card, say, at the end of yesterday?

CLIENT: Hmmm. Let me try to remember. Everything feels like such a blur. But last night, I remember I was at work late and when I got home my kid was needing a lot of attention. I didn't take any time for myself to sit down and fill out the diary card. I know it's in my best interest to fill it out, but I just didn't.

COTHERAPIST 2: My hunch is maybe that what you're describing is a pattern, with other demands interfering with what you think might be in your best interests.

CLIENT: It's definitely a pattern for me.

COTHERAPIST 1: So if this is indeed a pattern, one possibility is that certain emotions, possibly such as resentment, would build up as a result. Feelings that one might end up binge eating over. You put yourself off, put yourself off, put yourself off ... until you've had it. Not knowing how to regulate those emotions, you might end up relying on the binge to do it for you. Thinking about it now, what skill or skills that we've taught so far could help you at that moment? If you're not sure, ask the group for ideas.

Example 2: "I couldn't face doing homework."

CLIENT: I didn't fill out my diary card because I just didn't want to look at all this stuff. It felt too painful!

COTHERAPIST 1: This issue you're bringing up is very important. New patterns, such as putting yourself first in your life or getting yourself to face something you want to avoid—these are key if you're to stop binge eating.

CLIENT: I agree. Oddly, for some reason I was able to look at it this morning, and it wasn't bad at all. I actually kind of enjoyed it. So now I actually feel like doing it and regret that I didn't before.

COTHERAPIST 2: I can understand that regret. Maybe you feel like you missed out on something, on discovering something about yourself?

CLIENT: Yes. But I didn't want to know earlier.

COTHERAPIST 2: One of the things you're saying, and it really relates to what we talked about last session, is that when your mood and your behavior are tightly linked, if you don't feel like doing something, you can't follow through. Or, if you experience an urge to binge, this would mean that you have to binge. Regarding your homework, the question is how to manage the feelings of embarrassment, of not wanting to look at something that happened that day or something you did, while still following through on the behavior of completing your homework. We know that if you kind of give up and capitulate, you're opening yourself up to bingeing. Can you take a moment to think ahead to this coming week? What skills would help you to keep your awareness and focus? That's really the purpose of the daily forms, to help you be aware of what is going on.

Example 3: "I didn't understand how to fill out the chain analysis."

CLIENT: I got really confused and didn't understand how to do the chain. This kind of thing happens to me a lot. I look at things and think, "What am I supposed to be doing?" I'm very good at talking about my feelings, but writing them down is very difficult for me. And if I don't know, I deal with it by just closing the book.

COTHERAPIST 2: OK ... it's difficult but it is not impossible. One of the things that I think that you're describing, and we've seen in some other contexts, too, is capitulating. I'm just guessing, but there's probably some sort of judging about "Oh gosh, I can't figure this out exactly, I can't do it perfectly." Or maybe that it's too much, you won't be able to finish it all. So to manage the anxiety, you close the book and don't do any of it. I think you become overwhelmed by the judging.

CLIENT: I can fill out the diary card boxes daily. That seems more straightforward. But looking at the chain, I just think, how do I do this?

COTHERAPIST 1: You were able to do the diary card daily, that's terrific! And what you're doing right now is identifying some of the links that interfered with your filling out the chain. We are going to practice filling out the chain analysis later today in group, which should help. But I think one of the things that will be important for you is not to give up or expect that you will do it absolutely correctly, or that there even is a "right" or "perfect" way. Try to work with the chain as best you can. Break it into small blocks and tackle one block at a time. Even if you figure out a piece of it, complete one link or one of the boxes, that's a significant start.

Example 4: "I'll start to want to eat."

CLIENT: I looked at the blocks on the chain and said, "I can't do it. I'm just too overwhelmed. I'm going to start to want to eat." So I said, "forget it, I just won't do it." I sat and just relaxed. I said, "OK, I haven't done it. If they drop me out of the group, so be it." When I get overwhelmed I have to put whatever it is away and just take a deep breath.

COTHERAPIST 1: That can certainly be a very skillful thing to do. If you feel that your emotions are starting to become overwhelming or if they are building, it is very skillful to stop for a moment and take a rest. A key is to try to take a step back and center yourself with your breathing. We're going to talk more about that very skill today. The idea is that stepping back can actually help you find a way to do what would otherwise be overwhelming. You can maintain awareness without being fully caught up in your emotions.

CLIENT: I guess one thing I could do is to look at it again, after I've stopped and breathed.

COTHERAPIST 2: That makes sense—to check back in with yourself and, when you are ready, look at just one block, staying in close contact with yourself so you don't push yourself too hard.

CLIENT: I think I could.

In Session 2, the concept of dialectical abstinence was taught. The following vignette of an interaction between a group member and cotherapist highlights how the concept of dialectical abstinence can be applied.

CLIENT: Having binged "big time" today at an event I ran at work, I'm thinking it's too simplistic to think I can sit here and say to myself "I'm committed." I know there are skills you'll be teaching us, but I need to have those skills already so I'd know my commitment would have something to underpin it.

COTHERAPIST: Does it have to? Does a commitment have to be the same thing as the behavior? In other words, could you be committed to something wholly and not necessarily have the confidence that you could do it, not yet have the evidence that you could?

CLIENT: You could, but I always measure my commitment by my success. I'm achievement oriented.

COTHERAPIST: Think about the metaphor of Olympic athletes we were just talking about. Before they start the race, they are fully dedicated to going all out for the gold. If, after the race is over, they don't win it, then they deal as skillfully as they can with that. But when you're going for it, it can't be in your mind that "I can't say I'm committed to it because if I fail, then I'll be mad at myself" or

"I probably can't really do it" or "It's OK if I don't really do it." What we're saying is that it's important to your success to be able to hold two different things in your mind at the same time. One is the 100% commitment to yourself and to stopping binge eating. The other, which is not at the forefront of your mind, is the knowledge that if you do binge, you'll deal with it without beating yourself up. You'll pick yourself up, you'll learn from it, you'll say, "It's hard, I just started this program. I don't have all the skills yet" and then you're right back with "I'm 100% committed." This is dialectical abstinence.

CLIENT: I can catch a glimpse of what you're talking about when you put it that way.

COTHERAPIST: Great!

Core Mindfulness Module: Sessions 3–5

Urge Surfing

Though we have not had it occur often, sometimes a group member becomes emotionally dysregulated during the Urge Surfing exercise. Therapists can use this as an important opportunity to help the client to identify and practice her or his Emotion Regulation skills during the session.

COTHERAPIST: Would someone like to describe what it's like to Urge Surf with this malt ball?

CLIENT 1: (*Starts to cry.*) It's just too hard.

COTHERAPIST: I can really hear how upset you are (*gently*). Can you describe to me what emotion you're feeling right now?

CLIENT: All I can think about is binge eating. I'm okay while I'm here in the group but I'm upset because … (*sobs*) … after the session I'm just going to end up in the grocery store, and I'll buy more malt balls and more food. Maybe you had your reasons, but this was a terrible day for me to practice Urge Surfing. I wish I hadn't come to group.

CLIENT 2: I think this should stop. Can't you see she's really upset?

COTHERAPIST: (*Acknowledges that Client 2 has spoken but addresses Client 1.*) I know that you're feeling really distressed and wish you hadn't come to group today. Is that what you're feeling right now?

CLIENT 1: (*Gulps and nods.*)

COTHERAPIST: Maybe you could begin by taking a couple of breaths and just observe the sensations in your body.

CLIENT 1: I shouldn't cry in group.

COTHERAPIST: That sounds like a judgment, not a sensation (*teasingly*). Judgment duly noted, thank you for sharing.

CLIENT 1: (*Small giggle.*)

COTHERAPIST: OK, just let the judgment go. And tell me what you notice in your face, your chest. …

CLIENT 1: I can feel tears on my face, and they are wet. My chest is heavy.

COTHERAPIST: What are the thoughts and feelings that you're having right now?

CLIENT 1: I'm upset at myself for being upset right now in group. My husband always says I get upset too much and he can't cope with my feelings. I get too angry, too upset. Why can't I be normal?

COTHERAPIST: (*Gently but in a focused way.*) So what are your emotions right now?

CLIENT 1: I feel humiliated for crying in group.

COTHERAPIST: You mentioned an urge to go to the store after group to binge. What emotion do you think might be connected to that urge? Maybe anger at us for choosing to have you practice Urge Surfing today?

CLIENT 1: Well, right now I don't feel that any more. I just feel embarrassed.

CLIENT 2: I think you're showing heaps of courage in talking about how you're feeling right now.

CLIENT 1: I didn't feel like I had much choice, but thanks.

COTHERAPIST: So where is the urge to binge after group right now?

CLIENT 1: It's less. I think I can go on now.

Alternate Rebellion (Session 5)

Alternate Rebellion uses the Mindfulness "How" skill of Effectively to satisfy a client's wish to rebel without destroying her or his overriding objective of stopping binge eating. Although clients with BED relate easily to the concept behind the skill, we have found that they benefit from being given specific examples of how other clients from prior groups have put it into use.

> COTHERAPIST: "We really encourage you to be creative in using this skill. For example, some prior group members who felt judged by society for being overweight have 'rebelled' by buying a dessert, such as a single-serving ice cream cone, and eating it in public—in full view. Others have bought and worn beautiful lacy lingerie. One client was angry at her husband for buying doughnuts but not eating them himself. She poured salt on them and threw them in her backyard pool! (*Group members laugh.*) What are some ideas you have for using this skill?"

Emotion Regulation Module: Sessions 6–12

The following vignette illustrates the application of opposite action with a client who says he is feeling hopeless about treatment and does not want to practice the skills.

CLIENT 1: These skills don't work, and I don't think this treatment works. I've been coming here for almost three months, and last night I got into a big fight with the wife and downed a dozen doughnuts.

COTHERAPIST 1: When I hear doughnuts, I hear the opportunity for opposite action!

CLIENT 1: (*Laughing and groaning*) I knew you'd say something like that.

COTHERAPIST 1: I'm not saying that I don't hear how discouraged you are.

CLIENT: Yeah—I'm feeling hopeless. When I feel like this, I don't feel like practicing the skills or even coming here.

COTHERAPIST 1: How great that you practiced opposite action in coming here today. How can you practice opposite action next time you're faced with a fight with your wife and a dozen doughnuts?

CLIENT 1: What was the skill I practiced to get here today again?

COTHERAPIST 2: (*Laughing*) Hey, who remembers opposite action?

CLIENT 2: Opposite action is when you act opposite to the urge that goes with your emotion. It's good for when you want to change your mood. If you're depressed and your urge is to skip group and stay in bed, for example, acting opposite means getting out of bed and coming to group.

CLIENT 1: Oh, yeah, that's what I did today to get here! But when I'm angry at the wife, opposite action would mean practicing being nice even if I have the urge to yell.

COTHERAPIST 2: Right on!

CLIENT 1: (*Laughs.*) Well, it would have a better chance of helping than what I did!

COTHERAPIST 1: So do I have your commitment to practice this skill this week, whether or not you get in a fight, so you're ready in the future?

CLIENT 1: Can do.

Distress Tolerance Module: Sessions 13–18

The discussion of Radical Acceptance in a group session in particular can be difficult when clients challenge the skill by asserting that certain things are too awful to be accepted.

CLIENT: Radical Acceptance doesn't make sense for me.

COTHERAPIST: In what way don't you think it makes sense for you?

CLIENT: Because it means that if something awful has happened, then I have to be all OK about it. And there are some things that are too terrible to ever forgive. My mother gave me up to foster care, and I was treated terribly—I told her, but she didn't do anything. I can't forgive her for what she did to me, and I think about it all the time because it ruined my life.

COTHERAPIST: I'm so sorry that happened to you. You're making a really important point that we need to make sure is clear. Radically accepting something means accepting that a reality has occurred and recognizing its consequences. It doesn't require that you forgive your mother. Forgiveness is a choice and not a necessary outcome of Radical Acceptance. Practicing Radical Acceptance can help you deeply accept your emotions about your childhood. Then you can choose or not choose to forgive your mother. You might want to forgive if these emotions interfere with your quality of life. But a perfectly productive life is possible through Radical Acceptance without forgiveness. To deal with suffering, acceptance is all that's needed. Sometimes, just accepting your feelings as they are can make the suffering less.

Review of Skills and Planning for the Future: Sessions 19–20

In the last session, therapists had each group member read from their homework regarding their plans for the future.

COTHERAPIST 1: What are your plans for making sure that you practice the skills that have been so helpful to you?

CLIENT: I've made mini-copies of the diary card so I can carry it around in my purse. I've also gotten a new cover for my notebook with all my skills—bright red! So it will be really easy for me to spot!

COTHERAPIST 1: Wow—that's great. Tell me one difficult situation that kept coming up on your chains and what skills you will use to deal with it without using food.

CLIENT: I have the strongest urge to binge after dinner parties. I tend to skip most of the yummy foods when I'm there, like dessert, for instance, because I think I'm still overweight. But I get resentful when I leave and end up stopping at the grocery store. The skill I've gotten the most help from is Mindful Eating. I just need to remember to use it—that it's not the particular food that is a problem but using food to push down my feelings. Food itself is fine, and I can enjoy it for what it is I when I eat mindfully.

COTHERAPIST 1: That's terrific! Who would like to share next?

As noted in Chapter 7, group members often wish to mark the end of group with a ritual of some sort. We encourage group members to select a ritual they think most appropriate. In addition, we often distribute a list of quotes about emotions (Appendix 8.1).

Quotes about Emotions

Accepting does not necessarily mean "liking," "enjoying," or "condoning." I can accept what is—and be determined to evolve from there. It is not acceptance but denial that leaves me stuck.

—NATHANIEL BRANDEN

But are not this struggle and even the mistakes one may make better, and do they not develop us more, than if we kept systematically away from emotions?

—VINCENT VAN GOGH

Let's not forget that the little emotions are the great captains of our lives and we obey them without realizing it.

—VINCENT VAN GOGH

One's suffering disappears when one lets oneself go, when one yields—even to sadness.

—ANTOINE DE SAINT-EXUPÉRY
(translated from French by Curtis Cate)

Plenty of people miss their share of happiness, not because they never found it, but because they didn't stop to enjoy it.

—WILLIAM FEATHER

The impossible can always be broken down into possibilities.

—AUTHOR UNKNOWN

Once we accept our limits, we go beyond them.

—BRENDAN FRANCIS

CHAPTER 9

Future Directions

This chapter outlines several future directions for DBT for BED/BN. Our aim is to be expansive. While fully acknowledging the limited database from clinical trials, we believe it worthwhile to think more broadly about the implementation of DBT for eating disorders for future clinical and research endeavors. We first discuss modifications to the treatment for those working with adolescent clients. Second, we focus on reducing the risk of relapse after the formal end of treatment and enhancing the likelihood of maintaining abstinence. Third, we address including weight loss as a treatment target when working with obese clients. Fourth, we consider providing time-limited DBT for clients who have BED/BN and are concurrently being treated by clinicians without a background in treating eating disorders. Finally, we explore improving the cost-effectiveness of DBT for BED/BN.

WORKING WITH ADOLESCENT CLIENTS

Of relevance, adolescents with suicidal behaviors have been shown to be developmentally capable of responding to modified versions of DBT for BPD (Miller, Rathus, & Linehan, 2007). Given the lack of empirically supported treatments available for adolescents with eating disorders, it is important to investigate adapting existing treatments for adults with eating disorders to younger populations. Frequently, the first signs of an eating disorder become apparent during adolescence. Additionally, adolescence is synonymous with emotion dysregulation!

To date, limited preliminary evidence suggests that DBT for eating disorders can be usefully adapted for adolescents (Safer, Couturier, & Lock, 2007; Salbach-Andrae, Bohnekamp, Pfeiifer, Lehmkuhl, & Miller, 2008). Recently, Salbach-Andrae and colleagues (2008) described a case series of adolescents with anorexia and bulimia treated with 25 weeks of twice-weekly DBT (i.e., individual therapy and group skills training). Significant posttreatment improvements in eating-disorder behaviors and psychopathology symptoms were reported (Salbach-Andrae et al., 2008). In an earlier case report, Safer, Couturier, and Lock (2007) modified DBT for BED for a 16-year-old female binge eater. Their adolescent version of DBT for BED retained the majority of the treatment elements presented in this book's earlier chapters. For example, the behavioral chain analysis and diary card were unchanged. In addition, the format of sessions included homework review in the first part of the session, followed by the teaching of new skills. At the same time, as described next, a number of adolescent-specific modifications were introduced.

Modifications to the Introductory Sessions

The therapist met conjointly with the client and her parents for the first 15 minutes of the initial treatment orientation session, followed by a private meeting with the client. This provided an opportunity to introduce the parents and the client to an overall orientation to the DBT model, its goals, and the structure of treatment. Furthermore, it allowed discussion of the parents' role in treatment. Parents were told their responsibility would be to support their daughter as she attempted to generalize what she learned in therapy into her life, including her interactions with the family. If it became apparent that the parents could play a more direct role and that the client would like their help, the parents would be invited to attend sessions (lasting 30–60 minutes) following the patient's individual sessions. The specific number of these sessions would be decided based on clinical judgment. During those sessions, the client would be invited to teach her parents the skills she was learning in therapy, working with her parents to identify specific ways in which they could help her manage her feelings and behaviors more effectively.[1]

Modification to Distress Tolerance Skills: Sessions 2–5

Another modification used in this case report included changing the sequence of the skills taught. Distress Tolerance skills were introduced first based on the practical and concrete nature of these skills, felt to be more easily understood and utilized by adolescents and more likely to maintain their interest in treatment.

Modifications to Mindfulness Skills: Sessions 6–10

Extra sessions were added to this module based on experiences noted by Miller and colleagues (2007) in their work using DBT with suicidal adolescents. The concept of accessing one's Wise Mind can be challenging for adolescents, whose developmental stage includes identity formation and emotion identification. To address this challenge in DBT for BED/BN for adolescents, simpler, less abstract definitions were used to convey the Mindfulness concepts than those used with adults. Wise Mind was referred to as one's deepest "gut feeling" about the truth of the situation, and Emotion Mind as that "part of your mind whose advice totally depends on your current mood" (e.g., deciding that "I need a snack" must be the right course

---

[1]Whether the parents require separate skills training or are taught any necessary skills by the adolescent during the family session would be determined on a case-by-case basis.

of action when faced with a difficult homework problem instead of checking in more deeply with one's mind and body about what would truly be effective).

Alternate Rebellion was not modified for adolescents, though it is worth high-lighting this skill's particular salience for this population, many of whom are gradually exploring more independent thought processes and action patterns. This involves emphasizing the purpose of the skill, to find effective, adaptive means of regulating difficult feelings. Examples of ways adolescents may find it useful to practice Alternate Rebellion include the use of dress or fashion (e.g., by paint-ing fingers with garish nail polish, wearing loudly clashing colors, or redecorating their bedrooms).

Modification to Emotion Regulation Skills (Sessions 11–17)

A modification for adolescents in this module involved making the Adult Pleasant Events Schedule in the Linehan (1993b) skills manual relevant to teenagers. Items such as "thinking about retirement" were eliminated, and activities relevant to teens, such as "planning fun things to do during summer vacation," were added.

Addition of Interpersonal Effectiveness Skills (Sessions 18–21)

Interpersonal dilemmas are often of paramount importance to teens, and build-ing mastery in this area is a typical goal of adolescent development. Therefore, it seemed important to add this module when modifying the manual for adolescents. (Decreasing the number of review sessions allocated allowed the total number of sessions to be only slightly increased by this additional module, from 20 to 21.) Though it provided only preliminary corroboration for this modification, it is of interest that the client in the case report noted this module to be her most useful.

The interpersonal effectiveness skills, including focusing on the different types of desired outcomes (e.g., achieving one's objectives, preserving the relationship, maintaining self-respect), were taught and rehearsed using relevant age-appro-priate scenarios (e.g., requesting permission to attend a sleepover birthday party, obtaining parental permission to stay out late with friends).

Other Modifications for Adolescents

Homework was more frequently tackled collaboratively during sessions, at least initially. This was done to ensure understanding of the key concepts and to be considerate of academic demands on an adolescent attending school. Also, because adolescents are often hesitant to initiate calls to adults, the modified treatment involved scheduling between-session phone calls (so that the therapist expects the patient's call) and encouraging e-mail. Appropriate self-disclosure about the thera-pist's use of the skills in his or her life, as in DBT for BED/BN (and, of course, standard DBT) is always useful, but especially so with adolescents in lessening the adult–teen power differential and strengthening the alliance. Finally, role play-ing, with the therapist and patient switching roles, was an effective way for both patient and therapist to better appreciate the presence of differing points of view.

Familial Modifications

The most marked of the adolescent-specific modifications utilized by Safer and colleagues (2007) was the inclusion of family sessions as needed. In the case report (Safer et al., 2007), for example, 4 of the 21 sessions were expanded (by an extra 30–60 minutes) to include the adolescent's family. The justification was the consistent identification, via the chain analyses, of the client's sense of academic pressure being a trigger for her binge eating. Both the client and her family were highly achievement oriented, which is common in individuals with eating disorders. Bringing the subject of achievement into the open during family sessions, while also targeting it individually, allowed identification of a key dialectic for the family: accepting the teen just as she was while simultaneously wanting her to be as successful as possible. The client's perspective was validated, and she was encouraged to communicate more effectively with her parents about their expectations. This key dialectic is likely of relevance to other families with adolescents suffering from eating disorders. The client decreased her fears of failure without lowering her standards.

Interestingly, the use of the family as reinforcing agents appeared to be the most effective of the various interventions in the piloted case example. This may imply the existence of a common theme for parental involvement within treatments for adolescents with eating disorders, as suggested by the evidence pointing to the superior outcomes of family-based treatments for anorexia nervosa for those patients whose illness began before age 19 (Eisler et al., 1997; Robin et al., 1999; Russell, Szmukler, Dare, & Eisler, 1987).

IMPROVING MAINTENANCE OF ABSTINENCE/REDUCING RISK OF RELAPSE

Telch and colleagues (2001) reported a decrease in abstinence after DBT for BED, from 89% at posttreatment to 67% at 3-month follow-up to 56% at 6-month follow-up. In examining DBT for BN, Safer and colleagues (2001b) found that the frequency of binge eating and purging increased from posttreatment to 3-month follow-up. Clearly, the issue of improving maintenance among those initially responsive at posttreatment is important.

The following suggestions are as yet without empirical support but are presented as options for clinicians concerned about reducing relapse among clients who have received DBT for BED/BN treatment. These suggestions include (1) adding booster sessions; (2) providing online support; (3) offering ongoing advanced DBT for BED/BN groups; and (4) combining DBT with CBT or IPT.

Adding Booster Sessions

Clients may benefit from additional "booster" group sessions to aid in maintaining treatment gains made during therapy. The necessary frequency of such sessions is unclear. Because relapse in the Telch et al. studies (e.g., 2001) has been documented by the 3-month follow-up assessment, booster groups should likely begin meeting well before this point. Perhaps such groups might meet monthly, then bimonthly, decreasing in frequency over time. These sessions would focus on any problematic behaviors that clients have experienced occurring since their last meeting.

Rather than offering group sessions, another means of improving maintenance could include the option of treating clients individually after the completion of group treatment. A number of our clients have requested this, and in nonresearch settings it may be desirable for a number of reasons. Clients may feel that the group format moved at a pace ill suited to them and that they would benefit more from one-on-one treatment. Our experience is that some clients do indeed have difficulty making use of the group time. A stepped-care-type approach might involve identifying such clients during the group and offering them a course of individual treatment, with the possibility of rejoining a group that forms at a later time. The individual-session format may also be useful for clients who no longer have difficulties with binge eating but wish to apply their newly acquired emotion regulation skills to other quality-of-life targets (e.g., increasing their social support, starting to date, taking up new interests).

Providing Online and/or CD-ROM Support

Another option to improve treatment gains includes the development of support online and/or via CD-ROMs. Support might involve online chats between group members (possibly moderated by coleaders) and/or having group members fill out and submit online diary cards and chain analyses between group sessions while treatment is under way or as part of a booster session package. Other options include using personal digital assistants (PDAs) as a means of tracking. Preliminary findings for such innovative methods have been positive. For example, CBT for BED delivered by CD-ROM was reported to be a well-accepted and effective treatment modality (e.g., Shapiro et al., 2007). And in a study examining the role of Internet support versus face-to-face support in the maintenance of weight loss, no significant differences in weight loss were found (Harvey-Berino, Pintauro, Buzzel, & Gold, 2004).

Offering an Ongoing Advanced DBT for BED/BN Group

Maintenance might also be improved by offering clients an advanced DBT group after they have completed the 20-week DBT for BED/BN program as described. Rather than holding monthly booster sessions, this advanced group might meet weekly. Attendance could be allowed on a drop-in basis or through requiring commitment to a designated block of sessions.

Combining DBT with CBT or IPT

Given the different mechanisms hypothesized to underlie CBT, IPT, and DBT for BN or BED, research combining these treatments may enhance maintenance.

WORKING WITH OBESE CLIENTS
WHO HAVE BED—ADDING WEIGHT LOSS AS A TARGET

The DBT for BED and BN treatment as described focuses on helping clients achieve abstinence from binge eating, not on weight loss. After 20 sessions of DBT for BED, for example, clients had not lost significantly more weight than those assigned to a wait-list condition (Telch et al., 2001). The lack of influence on weight is consistent with that found in other BED treatments (e.g., Wilfley et al., 2002).

Numerous BED treatment studies have also indicated that participants who maintain abstinence from binge eating after treatment lose more than those who relapse (e.g., Agras, Telch, Arnow, Eldredge, & Marnell, 1997). Among clients with BED treated in the Telch et al. (2000, 2001) studies, for example, the mean weight loss after 20 group sessions was 4.2 pounds. At the 6-month follow-up assessment, those who maintained abstinence had lost an additional 7.2 pounds compared with an additional 1.5 pounds lost for those who relapsed (Safer, Lively, Telch, & Agras, 2002).

Given the prevalence of overweight and obesity among BED clients and the concomitant health concerns, the question of how to help such clients lose weight is of great significance. DBT for BED/BN, with its emotion regulation focus, might offer a unique option for obese clients if its skills were adapted to target the types of emotional dysregulation that lead clients to break their diets, to drop out of weight management and exercise programs, or to avoid weight loss attempts altogether. The suggestions (e.g., adapting the targeted problem behavior, combining DBT with other weight management treatments) offer preliminary directions for how such a weight management treatment might proceed when undertaken after the achievement of binge abstinence.

Adapting the Targeted Problem Behavior

As noted, DBT for BED/BN primarily targets reducing emotional eating behaviors such as binge eating, not reducing body weight. In other words, therapists would not label the consumption of high-calorie foods as a problem behavior if such foods were eaten mindfully and with control.

A weight-loss-oriented adaptation would include adapting the path to mindful eating (Chapter 3, Appendix 3.2). By adding additional targets, such as deviating from one's weight loss plan through overeating, high-calorie food choices, or physical inactivity (Figure 9.1), clients can conduct chain analyses on these behaviors. Such chain analyses would identify the particular emotions leading to lapses from the client's food plan. For example, if a client said he or she overate because he or she felt "deprived," the associated emotions and thoughts could be fully observed and described. This might involve observing the thoughts "The amount of food on my plate won't be enough" or "I won't be able to bear the hunger," accompanied by potential emotions such as fear or resentment. For clients who avoid engaging in physical activity because of shame, chain analyses could be used to explore what skills (e.g., opposite action) could be used in these situations.

PATH TO MINDFUL EATING

1. Stop any behavior that interferes with treatment.*

2. Stop binge eating—eating large or small amounts of food while experiencing a sense of loss of control.

3. Stop other problem behaviors—overeating, eating off plan, mindless eating, not exercising.

4. Decrease cravings, urges, preoccupation with food.

5. Decrease capitulating—that is, closing off options to not binge eat.

6. Decrease apparently irrelevant behaviors—for example, buying binge foods "for company"; scheduling a phone call during your exercise time.

FIGURE 9.1. Treatment targets. *Though not explicitly delineated in this model, decreasing any life-threatening behaviors takes precedence over the other targets, just as in standard DBT, if crises arise.

Combining DBT with Other Weight Management Treatments

DBT may be effectively combined with other weight management treatments such as bariatric surgery, BWL (including self-monitoring, nutrition education, exercise; e.g., Wing, 1998), appetite awareness therapy (Craighead, 2006; Hill, Craighead, Smith, & Safer, 2006), self-help (e.g., Weight Watchers), online weight loss programs, and antiobesity medication (e.g., orlistat, sibutramine).

CLIENTS WHO ARE CONCURRENTLY SEEING OTHER CLINICIANS WHO LACK BACKGROUND IN TREATING EATING DISORDERS

Clients participating in our research trials were restricted from receiving concurrent psychotherapy from outside clinicians. In other settings, however, it may be helpful to accept referrals from clinicians who do not have backgrounds in eating-disorder treatment and whose clients wish to receive a time-limited DBT for BED/BN treatment to focus on their eating-disorder behaviors. In such settings, the standard DBT case management strategy of consultation to the client would be used. In coaching clients to manage their relationship with another clinician, DBT therapists develop the client's sense of control and self-efficacy and reinforce the collegial nature of the therapist–client relationship.

IMPROVING DBT FOR BED/BN'S COST-EFFECTIVENESS

Treatment might be made more cost-effective by reducing the number of sessions. Instead of 20, as researched in the DBT for BED/BN trials (e.g., Safer et al., 2001b, in press; Telch et al., 2001), perhaps fewer sessions might deliver similar posttreatment results. Such shortened treatments may be particularly helpful for less symptomatic individuals, such as those meeting criteria for subthreshold BED or BN (e.g., binge eating and/or purging one time per week on average versus two times per week, as per DSM-IV-TR [American Psychiatric Association, 2000]). Other ways to increase cost-effectiveness include delivering treatment via a self-help format or online. Less expensive online prevention programs utilizing DBT skills to target individuals at risk for eating disorders should be considered.

It is hoped that this book's availability will enable other researchers to replicate and extend our work. The Appendix: Information for Researchers offers details on the criteria used for recruiting participants for our randomized trials, which assessments were administered, and the specific content taught (e.g., skills and worksheets) during each of the 20 research sessions.

APPENDIX

Information for Researchers

We have received multiple requests over the years for the treatment manual we developed and used in our research studies. This Appendix is intended to provide information, in a condensed format, on the criteria used for recruiting participants for our randomized trials, to outline the assessment instruments, and to detail the session-by-session therapeutic content (e.g., skills taught) and materials/handouts used.

INCLUSION AND EXCLUSION CRITERIA

Participants in the BED studies (Safer et al., in press; Telch et al., 2000, 2001) were required to meet full DSM-IV-TR research criteria (American Psychiatric Association, 2000). Those in the BN study (Safer et al., 2001b) were required to have had at least one binge–purge episode per week over the previous 3 months.[1]

Exclusionary criteria were (1) BMI < 17.5; (2) current suicidality or psychosis; (3) current drug or alcohol abuse; (4) concurrent participation in psychotherapy or weight loss treatment; (5) concurrent antidepressant or mood stabilizer use (Telch et al., 2001; Safer et al., 2001b) or less than 3 months of stable antidepressant dosages (Safer et al., in press); and (6) pregnancy or breastfeeding.

ASSESSMENTS

Participants were assessed at baseline, at completion of treatment, and at follow-up (e.g., 3 months, 6 months, 12 months).

The Eating Disorder Examination (EDE; Fairburn & Cooper, 1993) was administered to determine the diagnosis of BED, BN, or partial BN and to assess the frequency of binge and/or purge episodes.

---

[1]The rationale for using modified DSM-IV-TR criteria was to broaden the study's applicability. Commonly, patients seen in general clinic settings complain of considerable bulimic symptomatology, but, not meeting full criteria, they are often excluded from research. Eighty-one percent of the recruited participants met full DSM-IV-TR criteria for BN.

The Structured Clinical Interviews for DSM-IV (SCID-I and SCID-II; First, Spitzer, Gibbon, & Williams, 1995; First, Gibbon, Spitzer, Williams, & Benjamin, 1997) were used to assess current and lifetime Axis I and Axis II disorders at baseline. The Binge Eating Scale (BES; Gormally, Black, Daston, & Rardin, 1982) was included as a measure of the severity of binge-eating problems.

The Emotional Eating Scale (EES; Arnow et al., 1995) assesses the extent to which specific negative emotional states (e.g., anger, anxiety, and depression) prompt an individual to feel an urge to eat.

The Rosenberg Self-Esteem Scale (Rosenberg, 1979) measures beliefs and attitudes regarding general self-worth.

The Beck Depression Inventory (BDI; Beck, Ward, Mendelson, Mock, & Erbaugh, 1961) reports the degree of symptoms of depression.

The Positive and Negative Affect Schedule (PANAS; Watson, Clark, & Tellegen, 1988) asks individuals to report the extent to which they recently experienced positive and negative emotions.

The Negative Mood Regulation Scale (NMR; Catanzaro & Mearns, 1990) measures the participant's expectancy that a behavior or cognition will alleviate a negative mood state.

Weight and height were measured in lightweight clothing, with shoes removed.

SESSION-BY-SESSION CONTENT

Pretreatment Orientation

- Emotion Dysregulation Model of Problem Eating (Chapter 3, Appendix 3.1)
- Goals of Treatment, Goals of Skills Training, and Treatment Targets (Chapter 3, Appendix 3.2)
- Group Member, Individual Client, and Therapist Treatment Agreements (Chapter 3, Appendices 3.3–3.5)

Handouts Given at Each Session

Blank Diary Card (Chapter 3, Appendix 3.9)
Blank Chain Analysis (Chapter 3, Appendix 3.8)

Session 1

- Pros and cons of binge eating (and purging)
- Commitment to abstinence
- Review path to mindful eating
- Review Group Member and Therapist Agreements
- Orient clients to diary card (Chapter 3, Appendices 3.9–3.10), chain analysis (Chapter 3, Appendices 3.6–3.8)
- *Skills*: Commitment to abstinence, 3″ × 5″ card

Session 2

- Dialectical abstinence (Chapter 3, Appendix 3.13)
- Review chain analysis (Chapter 3, Appendices 3.11–3.12)
- *Skills*: Dialectical abstinence, diaphragmatic breathing

Mindfulness Core Module

Session 3

- Present three states of mind (Mindfulness Handout 1*; Chapter 4, Appendices 4.2–4.4)
- *Skills*: Wise Mind

Session 4

- "What" Skills (Mindfulness Handout 2*; "What Skills Homework Sheet, Chapter 4, Appendix 4.5)
- Mindful Eating exercise
- *Skills*: Observe, Describe, Participate, Mindful Eating

Session 5

- "How" Skills (Mindfulness Handout 3*; "How" Skills Homework Sheet, Chapter 4, Appendix 4.6)
- *Skills*: Nonjudgmental stance, One-Mindfully, Effectively, Urge Surfing (Urge Surfing (Homework Sheet, Chapter 4, Appendix 4.7), Alternate Rebellion (Alternate Rebellion Homework Sheet, Chapter 4, Appendix 4.7)

Emotion Regulation Module

Session 6

- Goals of Emotion Regulation (Emotion Regulation Handout 1)*
- Letting go of emotional suffering (Emotion Regulation Handout 9)*
- Primary and secondary emotions (Emotion Regulation Handout)*
- *Skills*: Mindfulness of Current Emotion, Loving Your Emotion

Session 7

- Model for Describing Emotions (Emotion Regulation Handout 3)*
- Ways to describe emotions (Emotion Regulation Handout 4)*
- Observe and describe emotions (Emotion Regulation Homework 1)*
- *Skills*: Identify Your Emotion(s)

Session 8

- Function of emotions (Emotion Regulation Handout 5)*
- Emotion diary (Emotion Regulation Homework 2)*
- *Skills*: Function of Emotion(s)

Session 9

- Reducing vulnerability to negative emotions (Emotion Regulation Handout 6)*
- Steps for increasing positive emotions (Emotion Regulation Handout 7)*

---

*For these handouts, see Linehan (1993b), *Skills Training Manual for Treating Borderline Personality Disorder.*

- Adult Pleasant Activities Schedule (Emotion Regulation Handout 8)*
- *Skills*: Reducing vulnerability, building mastery, building positive experiences, mindfulness of positive experiences

Session 10

- Changing emotions by acting opposite to the current emotion (Emotion Regulation Handout 10)*

Session 11

- Myths about emotions (Emotion Regulation Handout 2)*

Session 12

- Review of emotion regulation (review of all handouts)

Session 13

- Review of core mindfulness skills (review of all handouts)

Distress Tolerance Module

Session 14

- Orientation to Distress Tolerance (List of Distress Tolerance Skills to Be Taught, Chapter 6, Appendix 6.1)
- Guidelines for accepting reality: Observing Your Breath (Distress Tolerance Handout 2)*
- Distress Tolerance Homework Sheet 2*
- *Skills*: Observing your breath

Session 15

- Half-Smiling (Distress Tolerance Handout 3)*
- Awareness Exercises (Distress Tolerance Handout 4)*
- Distress Tolerance Homework Sheet 2*
- *Skills*: Half-smiling, Awareness Exercises

Session 16

- Orientation to acceptance skills—Radical Acceptance (Distress Tolerance Handout 5)*
- Burning Your Bridges (Chapter 6, Appendix 6.2)
- Distress Tolerance Homework Sheet 2*
- *Skills*: Radical Acceptance (Turning the Mind, Willingness), Burning Your Bridges

---

*For these handouts, see Linehan (1993b), *Skills Training Manual for Treating Borderline Personality Disorder*.

Session 17

- Crisis Survival skills
- Distress Tolerance Homework Sheet 1*
- *Skills*: Distract, Self-Soothe, Improve the Moment, Pros and Cons

Session 18

- Review of Distress Tolerance and skill strengthening (review of all handouts)

Session 19

- Review of Mindfulness, Emotion Regulation, Distress Tolerance
- Planning for the future (Planning for the Future Homework Sheet, Chapter 7, Appendix 7.1)
- *Skills*: Coping Ahead

Session 20

- Discuss future plans
- Good-byes

---

*For these handouts, see Linehan (1993b), *Skills Training Manual for Treating Borderline Personality Disorder.*

References

Abraham, S. F., & Beumont, P. J. (1982). How patients describe bulimia or binge eating. *Psychological Medicine, 12*, 625–635.

Agras, W. S., & Telch, C. F. (1998). The effect of caloric deprivation and negative affect on binge eating in obese binge-eating disordered women. *Behavior Therapy, 29*, 491–503.

Agras, W. S., Telch, C. F., Arnow, B., Eldredge, K., & Marnell, M. (1997). One-year follow-up of cognitive-behavioral therapy for obese individuals with binge eating disorder. *Journal of Consulting and Clinical Psychology, 65*, 343–347.

Agras, W. S., Telch, C. F., Arnow, B., Eldredge, K., Wilfley, D. E., Raeburn, S. D., et al. (1994). Weight-loss, cognitive-behavioral, and desipramine treatments in binge eating disorder: An additive design. *Behavior Therapy, 25*, 225–238.

Agras, W. S., Walsh, T., Fairburn, C. G., Wilson, G. T., & Kraemer, H. C. (2000). A multicenter comparison of cognitive-behavioral therapy and interpersonal psychotherapy for bulimia nervosa. *Archives of General Psychiatry, 57*, 459–466.

Althshuler, B. D., Dechow, P. C., Waller, D. A., & Hardy, B. W. (1990). An investigation of the oral pathologies occurring in bulimia nervosa. *International Journal of Eating Disorders, 9*, 191.

American Psychiatric Association. (2000). *Diagnostic and statistical manual of mental disorders* (4th ed., text rev.). Washington, DC: Author.

American Psychiatric Association. (2001). Practice guideline for the treatment of patients with borderline personality disorders. *American Journal of Psychiatry, 168*, 1–52.

Arnow, B., Kenardy, J., & Agras, W. S. (1992). Binge eating among the obese: A descriptive study. *Journal of Behavioral Medicine, 15*, 155–170.

Arnow, B., Kenardy, J., & Agras, W. S. (1995). The Emotional Eating Scale: The development of a measure to assess coping with negative affect by eating. *International Journal of Eating Disorders, 18*, 79–90.

Barley, W. D., Buie, S. E., Peterson, E. W., Hollingsworth, A. S., Griva, M., Hickerson, S. C., et al. (1993). Development of an inpatient cognitive-behavioral treatment program for borderline personality disorder. *Journal of Personality Disorders, 7*, 232–240.

Barlow, D. H., & Craske, M. G. (2007). *Mastery of your anxiety and panic: Client workbook* (4th ed.). New York: Oxford University Press.

Beck, A. T., Ward, C. H., Mendelson, M., Mock, J. E., & Erbaugh, J. K. (1961). An inventory for measuring depression. *Archives of General Psychiatry, 4*, 561–571.

Ben-Tovim, D. I., Walker, K., Gilchrist, P., Freeman, R., Kalucy, R., & Esterman, A. (2001). Outcome in patients with eating disorders: A 5-year study. *Lancet, 357*, 1254–1257.

Berkman, N. D., Lohr, K. N., & Bulik, C. M. (2007). Outcomes of eating disorders: A systematic review of the literature. *International Journal of Eating Disorders, 40*(4), 293–309.

Bohus, M., Haaf, B., & Simms, T. (2004). Effectiveness of inpatient dialectical behavior therapy for borderline personality disorder: A controlled trial. *Behaviour Research and Therapy, 42,* 487–499.

Bohus, M., Haaf, B., Stiglmayr, C., Pohl, U., Böhme, R., & Linehan, M. (2000). Evaluation of inpatient dialectical-behavioral therapy for borderline personality disorder: A prospective study. *Behaviour Research and Therapy, 38,* 875–887.

Brody, M. L., Walsh, B. T., & Devlin, M. J. (1994). Binge eating disorder: Reliability and validity of a new diagnostic category. *Journal of Consulting and Clinical Psychology, 62*(2), 381–386.

Bruce, B., & Agras, W. (1992). Binge eating in females: A population-based investigation. *International Journal of Eating Disorders, 12*(4), 365–373.

Bulik, C. M., Klump, K. L., Thornton, L., Kaplan, A. S., Devlin, B., Fichter, M. M., et al. (2004). Alcohol use disorder comorbidity in eating disorders: A multicenter study. *Journal of Clinical Psychiatry, 65,* 1000–1006.

Bulik, C. M., Lawson, R. H., & Carter, F. A. (1996). Salivary reactivity in restrained and unrestrained eaters and women with bulimia nervosa. *Appetite, 27,* 15–24.

Busetto, L., Segato, G., De Luca, M., De Marchi, F., Foletto, M., Vianello, M., et al. (2005). Weight loss and postoperative complications in morbidly obese patients with binge eating disorder treated by laparoscopic adjustable gastric banding. *Obesity Surgery, 15*(2), 195–201.

Casiero, D., & Frishman, W. H. (2006). Cardiovascular complications of eating disorders. *Cardiology in Review, 14,* 227–231.

Cassin, S. E., & von Ranson, K. M. (2005). Personality and eating disorders: A decade in review. *Clinical Psychology Review, 25,* 895–916.

Catanzaro, S. J., & Mearns, J. (1990). Measuring generalized expectancies for negative mood regulation: Initial scale development and implications. *Journal of Personality Assessment, 54,* 546–563.

Chambless, D. L., & Hollon, S. D. (1998). Defining empirically supported therapies. *Journal of Consulting and Clinical Psychology, 66,* 7–18.

Chen, E. Y., Matthews, L., Allen, C., Kuo, J., & Linehan, M. M. (2008). Dialectical behavior therapy for clients with binge-eating disorder or bulimia nervosa and borderline personality disorder. *International Journal of Eating Disorders, 41*(6), 505–512.

Chua, J. L., Touyz, S., & Hill, A. J. (2004). Negative mood-induced overeating in obese binge eaters: An experimental study. *International Journal of Obesity and Related Metabolic Disorders, 28,* 606–610.

Cialdini, R. B., Vincent, J. E., Lewis, S. K., Catalan, J., Wheeler, D., & Darby, B. L. (1975). Reciprocal concessions procedure for inducing compliance: The door-in-the-face technique. *Journal of Personality and Social Psychology, 31,* 206–215.

Cooper, Z., Cooper, P. J., & Fairburn, C. G. (1989). The validity of the Eating Disorder Examination and its subscales. *British Journal of Psychiatry, 154,* 806–812.

Corstorphine, E., Mountford, V., Tomlinson, S., Waller, G., & Meyer, C. (2007). Distress tolerance in the eating disorders. *Eating Behaviors, 8,* 91–97.

Craighead, L. W. (2006). *The appetite awareness workbook: How to listen to your body and overcome bingeing, overeating, and obsession with food.* Oakland, CA: New Harbinger.

de la Rie, S. M., Noordenbos, G., & van Furth, E. F. (2005). Quality of life and eating disorders. *Quality of Life Research: An International Journal of Quality of Life Aspects of Treatment, Care and Rehabilitation, 14,* 1511–1522.

de Zwaan, M., Mitchell, J. E., Howell, L. M., Monson, N., Swan-Kremeier, L., Crosby, R. D., et al. (2003). Characteristics of morbidly obese patients before gastric bypass surgery. *Comprehensive Psychiatry, 44,* 428–434.

Dobson, K. S., & Dozois, D. J. (2004). Attentional biases in eating disorders: A meta-analytic review of Stroop performance. *Clinical Psychology Review, 23,* 1001–1022.

Doll, H. A., Petersen, S. E., & Stewart-Brown, S. L. (2005). Eating disorders and emotional and physical well-being: Associations between student self-reports of eating disorders and quality of life as measured by the SF-26. *Quality of Life Research, 14,* 705–717.

Drewnowski, A., Yee, D. K., & Krahn, D. D. (1988). Bulimia in college women: Incidence and recovery rates. *American Journal of Psychiatry, 145,* 753–755.

Eisler, I., Dare, C., Russell, G. F., Szmukler, G., le Grange, D., & Dodge, E. (1997). Family and individual therapy in anorexia nervosa: A 5-year follow-up. *Archives of General Psychiatry, 54,* 1025–1030.

Eldredge, K. L., & Agras, W. S. (1996). Weight and shape overconcern and emotional eating in binge eating disorder. *International Journal of Eating Disorders, 19,* 73–82.

Fairburn, C. G. (1995). *Overcoming binge eating.* New York: Guilford Press.

Fairburn, C. G., & Brownell, K. D. (Eds.). (2001). *Eating disorders and obesity* (2nd ed.). New York: Guilford Press.

Fairburn, C. G., & Cooper, Z. (1993). The Eating Disorder Examination (12th ed.). In C. G. Fairburn & G. T. Wilson (Eds.), *Binge eating: Nature, assessment, and treatment* (pp. 317–360). New York: Guilford Press.

Fairburn, C. G., Cooper, Z., Doll, H. A., Norman, P., & O'Connor, M. (2000). The natural course of bulimia nervosa and Binge Eating Disorder in young women. *Archives of General Psychiatry, 57,* 659–665.

Fichter, M. M., Quadflieg, N., & Hedlund, S. (2008). Long-term course of binge eating disorder and bulimia nervosa: Relevance for nosology and diagnostic criteria. *International Journal of Eating Disorders, 41,* 577–586.

First, M. B., Gibbon, M., Spitzer, R. L., Williams, J. B. W., & Benjamin, L. S. (1997). *Structured clinical interview for DSM-IV Axis II disorders (SCID-II).* Washington, DC: American Psychiatric Press.

First, M. B., Spitzer, R. L., Gibbon, M., & Williams, J. B. W. (1995). *Structured clinical interview for DSM-IV Axis I disorders—Patient edition* (SCID-I/P, version 2.0). New York: New York State Psychiatric Institute, Biometrics Research Department.

Freedman, J. L., & Fraser, S. C. (1966). Compliance without pressure: The foot-in-the-door technique. *Journal of Personality and Social Psychology, 57,* 195–202.

Garner, D. M., & Garfinkel, P. E. (1997). *Handbook of treatment for eating disorders* (2nd ed.). New York: Guilford Press.

Godart, N. T., Perdereau, F., Rein, Z., Berthoz, S., Wallier, J., Jeammet, P., et al. (2007). Comorbidity studies of eating disorders and mood disorders. Critical review of the literature. *Journal of Affective Disorders, 97,* 37–49.

Goldstein, J., & Kornfield, J. (1987). *Seeking the heart of wisdom: The pattern of insight mediation.* Boston: Shambhala.

Gormally, J., Black, S., Daston, S., & Rardin, D. (1982). The assessment of binge eating severity among obese persons. *Addictive Behaviors, 7,* 47–55.

Greeno, C. G., Wing, R. R., & Shiffman, S. (2000). Binge antecedents in obese women with and without binge eating disorder. *Journal of Consulting and Clinical Psychology, 68,* 95–102.

Grilo, C. M., Sanislow, C. A., Shea, M. T., Skodol, A. E., Stout, R. L., Pagano, M. E., et al. (2003). The natural course of bulimia nervosa and eating disorders not otherwise specified is not influenced by personality disorders. *International Journal of Eating Disorders, 34* 319–330.

Gross, J. J. (Ed.). (2006). *Handbook of emotion regulation.* New York: Guilford Press.

Hanh, T. N. (1999). *The miracle of mindfulness: A Manual of Meditation.* Boston: Beacon Press.

Hansel, S., & Wittrock, D. A. (1997). Appraisal and coping strategies in stressful situations: A comparison of individuals who binge eat and controls. *International Journal of Eating Disorders, 21,* 89–93.

Harvey-Berino, J., Pintauro, S., Buzzell, P., & Gold, E. C. (2004). Effect of Internet support on the long-term maintenance of weight loss. *Obesity Research, 12,* 320–329.

Healy, K., Conroy, R. M., & Walsh, N. (1985). The prevalence of binge-eating and bulimia in 1,063 college students. *Journal of Psychiatric Research, 19,* 161–166.

Herzog, D. B., Dorer, D. J., Keel, P. K., Selwyn, S. E., Ekeblad, E. R., Flores, A. T., et al. (1999). Recovery and relapse in anorexia and bulimia nervosa: A 7.5-year follow-up study. *Journal of the American Academy of Child and Adolescent Psychiatry, 38,* 829–837.

Herzog, D. B., Franko, D. L., Dorer, D. J., Keel, P. K., Jackson, S., & Manzo, M. P. (2006). Drug abuse in women with eating disorders. *International Journal of Eating Disorders, 39,* 364–368.

Herzog, D. B., Keller, M. B., Lavori, P. W., & Ott, I. L. (1987). Social impairment in bulimia. *International Journal of Eating Disorders, 6,* 741–747.

Hill, D. M., Craighead, L. W., Smith, L., & Safer, D. L. (2006, November). *Appetite-focused DBT for the treatment of binge eating and purging: A preliminary report.* Poster session presented at the meeting of the Association for Behavioral and Cognitive Therapies, Chicago.

Hoek, H. W., & van Hoeken, D. (2003). Review of the prevalence and incidence of eating disorders. *International Journal of Eating Disorders, 34,* 383–396.

Hsu, L. K. (1996). "Epidemiology of the eating disorders." *Psychiatric Clinics of North America, 19,* 681–700.

Hsu, L. K., Betancourt, S., & Sullivan, S. P. (1996). Eating disturbances before and after vertical banded gastroplasty: A pilot study. *International Journal of Eating Disorders, 19,* 23–34.

Hsu, L. K. G., Mulliken, B., McDonagh, B., Krupa

Das, S. K., Rand, W., Fairburn, C. G., et al. (2002). Binge eating disorder in extreme obesity. *International Journal of Obesity, 26*(10), 1398–1403.

Hsu, L. K., Sullivan, S. P., & Benotti, P. N. (1997). Eating disturbances and outcome of gastric bypass surgery: A pilot study. *International Journal of Eating Disorders, 21*, 385–390.

Johnson, C., & Larson, R. (1982). Bulimia: An analysis of moods and behavior. *Psychosomatic Medicine, 44*, 341–351.

Kabat-Zinn, J. (1990). *Full catastrophe living.* New York: Dell.

Kaplan, A. S., & Garfinkel, P. E. (Eds.). (1993). *Medical issues and the eating disorders: The interface.* New York: Brunner/Mazel.

Katzman, M. A., & Wolchik, S. A. (1984). Bulimia and binge eating in college women: A comparison of personality and behavioral characteristics. *Journal of Consulting and Clinical Psychology, 52*, 423–428.

Keel, P. K., & Mitchell, J. E. (1997). Outcome in bulimia nervosa. *American Journal of Psychiatry, 154*, 313–321.

Keel, P. K., Mitchell, J. E., Miller, K. B., Davis, T. L., & Crow, S. J. (2000). Social adjustment over 10 years following diagnosis with bulimia nervosa. *International Journal of Eating Disorders, 27*, 21–28.

Kenardy, J., Mensch, M., Bowen, K., & Dalton, M. (2001). Disordered eating in Type 2 diabetes. *Eating Behavior, 2*, 183–192.

Kenardy, J., Mensch, M., Bowen, K., & Pearson, S. (1994). A comparison of eating behaviors in newly diagnosed non-insulin-dependent diabetes mellitus and case-matched controls. *Diabetes Care, 17*, 1197–1199.

Kessler, R. C., Berglund, P., Demler, O., Jin, R., Koretz, D., Merikangas, K. R., et al. (2003). The epidemiology of major depressive disorder: Results from the National Comorbidity Survey Replication (NCS-R). *Journal of the American Medical Association, 289*, 3095–3105.

Kessler, R. C., Berglund, P., Demler, O., Jin, R., Merikangas, K. R., & Walters, E. E. (2005). Lifetime prevalence and age-of-onset distributions of DSM-IV disorders in the National Comorbidity Survey Replication. *Archives of General Psychiatry, 62*, 593–602.

Klerman, G. L., & Weissman, M. M. (Eds.). (1993). *New applications of interpersonal therapy.* Washington, DC: American Psychiatric Press.

Koons, C. R., Robins, C. J., Tweed, J. L., Lynch, T. R., Gonzalez, A. M., Morse, J. Q., et al. (2001). Efficacy of dialectical behavior therapy in women veterans with borderline personality disorder. *Behavior Therapy, 32*, 371–390.

Lacey, J. H. (1993). Self-damaging and addictive behaviour in bulimia nervosa: A catchment area study. *British Journal of Psychiatry, 163*, 190–194.

Laird, J. D. (1974). Self-attribution of emotion: The effects of expressive behavior on the quality of emotional experience. *Journal of Personality and Social Psychology, 29*, 475–486.

Legenbauer, T., Vocks, S., & Rüddel, H. (2008). Emotion recognition, emotional awareness and cognitive bias in individuals with bulimia nervosa. *Journal of Clinical Psychology, 64*, 687–702.

Lieb, K., Zanarini, M. C., Schmahl, C., Linehan, M. M., & Bohus M. (2004). Borderline personality disorder. *Lancet, 364*, 453–461.

Linehan, M. M. (1993a). *Cognitive-behavioral treatment of borderline personality disorder.* New York: Guilford Press.

Linehan, M. M. (1993b). *Skills training manual for treating borderline personality disorder.* New York: Guilford Press.

Linehan, M. M., Armstrong, H. E., Suarez, A., Allmon, D., & Heard, H. L. (1991). Cognitive-behavioral treatment of chronically parasuicidal borderline patients. *Archives of General Psychiatry, 48*, 1060–1064.

Linehan, M. M., & Chen, E. Y. (2005). Dialectical behavior therapy for eating disorders. In A. Freeman (Ed.), *Encyclopedia of cognitive behavior therapy* (pp. 168–171). New York: Springer.

Linehan, M. M., Comtois, K., Brown, M., Reynolds, S., Welch, S., Sayrs, J., et al. (2002, November). *DBT versus nonbehavioral treatment by experts in the community: Clinical outcomes.* Symposium presentation for the Association for Advancement of Behavior Therapy, Reno, NV.

Linehan, M. M., Comtois, K. A., Murray, A. M., Brown, M. Z., Gallop, R. J., Heard, H. L., et al. (2006). Two-year randomized controlled trial and follow-up of dialectical behavior therapy vs. therapy by experts for suicidal behaviors and borderline personality disorder. *Archives of General Psychiatry, 63*(7), 757–766.

Linehan, M. M., & Dimeff, L. A. (1997). *Dialectical behavior therapy manual of treatment interventions for drug abusers with borderline personality disorder.* Seattle, WA: University of Washington.

Linehan, M. M., Dimeff, L. A., Reynolds, S. K., Comtois, K. A., Welch, S. S., Heagerty, P., et al. (2002). Dialectical behavior therapy versus comprehensive validation therapy plus 12-step for the treatment of opioid dependent women meeting criteria for borderline personality disorder. *Drug and Alcohol Dependence, 67*(1), 13–26.

Linehan, M. M., Heard, H. L., & Armstrong, H. E. (1993). Naturalistic follow-up of a behavioral treatment for chronically parasuicidal borderline patients. *Archives of General Psychiatry, 50*, 971–974.

Linehan, M. M., Schmidt, H., III, Dimeff, L. A., Craft, J. C., Kanter, J., & Comtois, K. A. (1999). Dialectical behavior therapy for patients with borderline personality disorder and drug dependence. *American Journal of Addiction, 8*, 279–292.

Linehan, M. M., Tutek, D. A., Heard, H. L., & Armstrong, H. E. (1994). Interpersonal outcome of cognitive behavioral treatment for chronically suicidal borderline patients. *American Journal of Psychiatry, 151*, 1771–1776.

Lingswiler, V. M., Crowther, J. H., & Stephens, M. A. (1987). Emotional reactivity and eating in binge eating and obesity. *Journal of Behavioral Medicine, 10*, 287–299.

Lingswiler, V. M., Crowther, J. H., & Stephens, M. A. (1989). Affective and cognitive antecedents to eating episodes in bulimia and binge eating. *International Journal of Eating Disorders, 8*(5), 533–539.

Lynch, W. C., Everingham, A., Dubitzky, J., Harman, M., & Kassert, T. (2000). Does binge eating play a role in the self-regulation of moods? *Integrative Physiological and Behavioral Science, 35*(4), 298–313.

Marcus, M. D. (1997). Adapting treatment for patients with binge-eating disorder. In D. M. Garner & P. R. Garfinkel (Eds.), *Handbook of treatment for eating disorders* (2nd ed., pp. 484–493). New York: Guilford Press.

Marcus, M. D., Wing, R. R., & Fairburn, C. G. (1995). Cognitive behavioral treatment of binge eating vs. behavioral weight control on the treatment of binge eating disorder. *Annals of Behavioral Medicine, 17*, S090.

Marlatt, G. A. (1994). Addiction, mindfulness, and acceptance. In S. C. Hayes, N. S. Jacobson, V. M., Follette, & M. J. Dougher (Eds.), *Acceptance and change: Content and context in psychotherapy* (pp. 175–197). Reno, NV: Content Press.

Masheb, R. M., & Grilo, C. M. (2006). Emotional overeating and its associations with eating disorder psychopathology among overweight patients with binge eating disorder. *International Journal of Eating Disorders, 39*, 141–146.

Mauler, B. I., Hamm, A. O., Weike, A. I., & Tuschen-Caffier, B. J. (2006). Affect regulation and food intake in bulimia nervosa: Emotional responding to food cues after deprivation and subsequent eating. *Abnormal Psychology, 115*, 567–579.

McCabe, E. B., La Via, M. C., & Marcus, M. D. (2004). Dialectical behavior therapy for eating disorders. In J. K. Thompson (Ed.), *Handbook of eating disorders and obesity* (pp. 232–244). New York: Wiley.

McCann, R. A., Ball, E. M., & Ivanoff, A. (2000). DBT with an inpatient forensic population: The CMHIP forensic model. *Cognitive and Behavioral Practice, 7*, 447–456.

Mehler, P. S., Crews, C., & Weiner, K. (2004). Bulimia: Medical complications. *Journal of Women's Health, 13*(6), 668–675.

Miller, A. L., Rathus, J. H., & Linehan, M. M. (2007). *Dialectical behavior therapy with suicidal adolescents*. New York: Guilford Press.

Milos, G., Spindler, A., Schnyder, U., & Fairburn, C. G. (2005). Instability of eating disorder diagnoses: Prospective study. *British Journal of Psychiatry, 187*, 573–578.

Mitchell, J. E., & Crow, S. (2006). Medical complications of anorexia nervosa and bulimia nervosa. *Current Opinion in Psychiatry, 19*, 438–443.

Mitchell, J. E., Hatsukami, D., Eckert, E. D., & Pyle, R. I. (1985). Characteristics of 275 patients with bulimia. *American Journal of Psychiatry, 142*, 482–485.

Munsch, S., Biedert, E., Meyer, A., Michael, T., Schlup, B., Tuch, A., et al. (2007). A randomized comparison of cognitive behavioral therapy and behavioral weight loss treatments for overweight individuals with binge eating disorder. *International Journal of Eating Disorders, 40*, 102–113.

National Heart, Lung, and Blood Institute, and NHLBI Obesity Education Initiative Expert Panel. (1998). Clinical guidelines on the identification, evaluation, and treatment of overweight and obesity in adults: The evidence report. *Obesity Research, 6*(Suppl. 2), S51–S209.

Niego, S. H., Kofman, M. D., Weiss, J. J., & Geliebter, A. (2007). Binge eating in the bariatric surgery population: A review of the literature.

International Journal of Eating Disorders, 40, 349–359.

Pagoto, S., Bodenlos, J. S., Kantor, L., Gitkind, M., Curtin, C., & Ma, Y. (2007). Association of major depression and binge eating disorder with weight loss in a clinical setting. *Obesity, 15,* 2557–2559.

Palmer, R. L., Birchall, H., Damani, S. Gatward, N., McGrain, L., & Parker, L. (2003). A dialectical behavior therapy program for people with an eating disorder and borderline personality disorder: Description and outcome. *International Journal of Eating Disorders, 33,* 281–286.

Pi-Sunyer, F. X. (2002). The obesity epidemic: Pathophysiology and consequences of obesity. *Obesity Research, 10*(Suppl. 2), 975S–1045S.

Picot, A. K., & Lilenfeld, R. R. (2003). The relationship among binge severity, personality psychopathology, and body mass index. *International Journal of Eating Disorders, 34,* 98–107.

Polivy, J., & Herman, C. (1993). Etiology of binge eating: Psychological mechanisms. In C. G. Fairburn & G. T. Wilson (Eds.), *Binge eating: Nature, assessment, and treatment* (pp. 173–205). New York: Guilford Press.

Powell, A. L., & Thelen, M. H. (1996). Emotions and cognitions associated with bingeing and weight control behavior in bulimia. *Journal of Psychosomatic Research, 40*(3), 317–328.

Pyle, R., Halvorson, P., Neuman, P., & Mitchell, J. (1986). The increasing prevalence of bulimia in freshman college students. *International Journal of Eating Disorders, 52,* 631–647.

Pyle, R., Neuman, P., Halvorson, P., & Mitchell, J. (1991). An ongoing cross-sectional study of the prevalence of eating disorders in freshman college students. *International Journal of Eating Disorders, 10,* 667–677.

Rathus, J. H., & Miller, A. L. (2002). Dialectical behavior therapy adapted for suicidal adolescents. *Suicide and Life-Threatening Behavior, 32,* 146–157.

Rieger, E., Schotte, D. E., Touyz, S. W., Beumont, P. J., Griffiths, R., & Russell, J. (1998). Attentional biases in eating disorders: A visual probe detection procedure. *International Journal of Eating Disorders, 23,* 199–205.

Rieger, E., Wilfley, D. E., Stein, R. I., Marino, V., & Crow, S. J. (2005). A comparison of quality of life in obese individuals with and without binge eating disorder. *International Journal of Eating Disorders, 37*(3), 234–240.

Robin, A. L., Siegel, P. T., Moye, A. W., Gilroy,

M., Dennis, A. B., & Sikand, A. (1999). A controlled comparison of family versus individual therapy for adolescents with anorexia nervosa. *Journal of the American Academy of Child and Adolescent Psychiatry, 38,* 1428–1489.

Rorty, M., Yager, J., Buckwalter, J. G., & Rossotto, E. (1999). Social support, social adjustment, and recovery status in bulimia nervosa. *International Journal of Eating Disorders, 26*(1), 1–12.

Rosenberg, M. (1979). *Conceiving the self.* New York: Basic Books.

Russell, G. F., Szmukler, G. I., Dare, C., & Eisler, I. (1987). An evaluation of family therapy in anorexia nervosa and bulimia nervosa. *Archives of General Psychiatry, 44,* 1047–1056.

Rydall, A. C., Rodin, G. M., Olmsted, M. P., Devenyi, R. G., & Daneman, D. (1997). Disordered eating behavior and microvascular complications in young women with insulin-dependent diabetes mellitus. *New England Journal of Medicine, 336,* 1849–1854.

Safer, D. L., Couturier, J. L., & Lock, J. (2007). Dialectical behavior therapy modified for adolescent binge eating disorder: A case report. *Cognitive and Behavioral Practice, 14,* 157–167.

Safer, D. L., Lively, T. J., Telch, C. F., & Agras, W. S. (2002). Predictors of relapse following successful therapy for binge eating disorder. *International Journal of Eating Disorders, 32,* 155–163.

Safer, D. L., Robinson, A. H., & Jo, B. (in press). Outcome from a randomized controlled trial of group therapy for binge-eating disorder: Comparing dialectical behavior therapy adapted for binge eating to an active comparison group therapy. *Behavior Therapy.*

Safer, D. L., Telch, C. F., & Agras, W. S. (2001a). Dialectical behavior therapy adapted for bulimia: A case report. *International Journal of Eating Disorders, 30,* 101–106.

Safer, D. L., Telch, C. F., & Agras, W. S. (2001b). Dialectical behavior therapy for bulimia nervosa. *American Journal of Psychiatry, 158,* 632–634.

Salbach, H., Klinkowski, N., Pfeiffer, E., Lehmkuhl, U., & Korte, A. (2007). Dialectical behavior therapy for adolescents with anorexia and bulimia nervosa (DBT-AN/BN): A pilot study. *Praxis der Kinderpsychologie und Kinderpsychiatrie, 56,* 91–108.

Salbach-Andrae, H., Bohnekamp, I., Pfeiffer, E., Lehmkuhl, U., & Miller, A. L. (2008).

Dialectical behavior therapy of anorexia and bulimia nervosa among adolescents: A case series. *Cognitive and Behavioral Practice, 15,* 415–425.

Sallet, P. C., Sallet, J. A., Dixon, J. B., Collis, E., Pisani, C. E., Levy, A., et al. (2007). Eating behavior as a prognostic factor for weight loss after gastric bypass. *Obesity Surgery, 17,* 445–451.

Samuels, J., Eaton, W. W., Bienvenu, O. J., Brown, C. H., Costa, P. T., & Nestadt, G. (2002). Prevalence and correlates of personality disorders in a community sample. *British Journal of Psychiatry, 180,* 536–542.

Sansone, R. A., & Sansone, L. A. (1994). Bulimia nervosa: Medical complications. In L. Alexander-Mott & D. B. Lumsden (Eds.), *Understanding eating disorders: anorexia nervosa, bulimia nervosa, and obesity* (pp. 181–201). Washington, DC: Taylor & Francis.

Schotte, D. E., McNally, R. J., & Turner, M. L. (1990). A dichotic listening analysis of body weight concern in bulimia nervosa. *International Journal of Eating Disorders, 9,* 109–113.

Shapiro, J. R., Reba-Harrelson, L., Dymek-Valentine, M., Woolson, S. L., Hamer, R. M., & Bulik, C. M. (2007). Feasibility and acceptability of CD-ROM-based cognitive-behavioural treatment for binge-eating disorder. *European Eating Disorders Review, 15,* 175–184.

Smyth, J. M., Wonderlich, S. A., Heron, K. E., Sliwinski, M. J., Crosby, R. D., Mitchell, J. E., et al. (2007). Daily and momentary mood and stress are associated with binge eating and vomiting in bulimia nervosa patients in the natural environment. *Journal of Consulting and Clinical Psychology, 75,* 629–638.

Specker, S., de Zwaan, M., Raymond, N., & Mitchell, J. (1994). Psychopathology in subgroups of obese women with and without binge eating disorder. *Comprehensive Psychiatry, 35,* 185–190.

Spitzer, R. L., Devlin, M., Walsh, B. T., Hasin, D., Wing, R., Marcus, M. D., et al. (1992). Binge eating disorder: A multisite field trial of the diagnostic criteria. *International Journal of Eating Disorders, 11*(3), 191–203.

Spitzer, R. L., Yanovski, S., Wadden, T., Wing, R., Marcus, M. D., Stunkard, A., et al. (1993). Binge eating disorder: Its further validation in a multisite study. *International Journal of Eating Disorders, 13*(2), 137–153.

Spurrell, E. B., Wilfley, D. E., Tanofsky, M. B., & Brownell, K. D. (1997). Age of onset for binge eating: Are there different pathways to binge eating? *International Journal of Eating Disorders, 21,* 55–65.

Stanley, B., Ivanoff, A., Brodsky, B., Oppenheim, S., & Mann, J. (1998, November). Comparison of DBT and "treatment as usual" in suicidal and self-mutilating behavior. Paper presented at the Association for the Advancement of Behavior Therapy Convention, Washington, DC.

Steiger, H., Gauvin, L., Engelberg, M. J., Kin, N. M., Israel, M., Wonderlich, S., et al. (2005). Mood- and restraint-based antecedents to binge episodes in bulimia nervosa: Possible influences of the serotonin system. *Psychological Medicine, 35,* 1553–1562.

Stice, E., Killen, J. D., Hayward, C., & Taylor, C. B. (1998). Age of onset for binge eating and purging during late adolescence: A 4-year survival analysis. *Journal of Abnormal Psychology, 107,* 671–675.

Stickney, M. I., Miltenberger, R. G., & Wolff, G. (1999). A descriptive analysis of factors contributing to binge eating. *Journal of Behavior Therapy and Experimental Psychiatry, 30,* 177–189.

Swinbourne, J. M., & Touyz, S. W. (2007). The co-morbidity of eating disorders and anxiety disorders: A review. *European Eating Disorder Review, 15,* 253–274.

Telch, C. F. (1997a). *Emotion regulation skills training treatment for binge eating disorder: Therapist manual.* Unpublished manuscript, Stanford University.

Telch, C. F. (1997b). Skills training treatment for adaptive affect regulation in a woman with binge-eating disorder. *International Journal of Eating Disorders, 22*(1), 77–81.

Telch, C. F., & Agras, W. S. (1994). Obesity, binge eating and psychopathology: Are they related? *International Journal of Eating Disorders, 15,* 53–61.

Telch, C. F., & Agras, W. S. (1996). Do emotional states influence binge eating in the obese? *International Journal of Eating Disorders, 20,* 271–279.

Telch, C. F., Agras, W. S., & Linehan, M. M. (2000). Group dialectical behavior therapy for binge-eating disorder: A preliminary, uncontrolled trial. *Behavior Therapy, 31,* 569–582.

Telch, C. F., Agras, W. S., & Linehan, M. M. (2001). Dialectical behavior therapy for binge eating disorder. *Journal of Consulting and Clinical Psychology, 69*(6), 1061–1065.

Telch, C. F., Agras, W. S., & Rossiter, E. M.

(1988). Binge eating increases with increasing adiposity. *International Journal of Eating Disorders, 7*, 115–119.

Telch, C. F., & Stice, E. (1998). Psychiatric comorbidity in women with binge eating disorder: Prevalence rates from a non-treatment-seeking sample. *Journal of Consulting and Clinical Psychology, 66*, 768–776.

Turner, R. M. (2000). Naturalistic evaluation of dialectical behavior therapy-oriented treatment for borderline personality disorder. *Cognitive and Behavioral Practice, 7*, 413–419.

Verheul, R., Van Den Bosch, L. M., Koeter, M. W., De Ridder, M. A., Stijnen, T., & Van Den Brink, W. (2003). Dialectical behaviour therapy for women with borderline personality disorder: 12-month, randomised clinical trial in the Netherlands. *British Journal of Psychiatry, 182*, 135–140.

Waller, G. (2003). The psychology of binge eating. In C. G. Fairburn & K. D. Brownell (Eds.), *Eating disorders and obesity: A comprehensive handbook* (2nd ed., pp. 98–107). New York: Guilford Press.

Waller, G., Babbs, M., Milligan, R., Meyer, C., Ohanian, V., & Leung, N. (2003). Anger and core beliefs in the eating disorders. *International Journal of Eating Disorders, 34*, 118–124.

Watson, D., Clark, L., & Tellegen, A. (1988). Development and validation of brief measures of positive and negative affect: The PANAS scales. *Journal of Personality and Social Psychology, 54*, 1063–1070.

Whiteside, U., Chen, E. Y., Neighbors, C., Hunter, D., Lo, T., & Larimer, M. (2007). Difficulties regulating emotions: Do binge eaters have fewer strategies to modulate and tolerate negative affect? *Eating Behaviors, 8*, 162–169.

Wilfley, D. E., Agras, W. S., Telch, C. F., Rossiter, E. M., Schneider, J. A., Cole, A. G., et al. (1993). Group cognitive-behavioral therapy and group interpersonal psychotherapy for the nonpurging bulimic individual: A controlled comparison. *Journal of Consulting and Clinical Psychology, 61*, 296–305.

Wilfley, D. E., Welch, R. R., Stein, R. I., Spurrell, E. B., Cohen, L. R., Saelens, B. E., et al. (2002). A randomized comparison of group cognitive-behavioral therapy and group interpersonal therapy for the treatment of overweight individuals with binge eating disorder. *Archives of General Psychiatry, 59*, 713–721.

Wilson, G. T., Fairburn, C. G., & Agras, W. S. (1997). Cognitive-behavioral therapy for bulimia nervosa. In D. M. Garner & P. E. Garfinkel (Eds.), *Handbook of treatment for eating disorders* (2nd ed., pp. 67–93). New York: Guilford Press.

Wilson, G. T., Grilo, C. M., & Vitousek, K. M. (2007). Psychological treatment of eating disorders. *American Psychologist, 62*, 199–216.

Wilson, G. T., Nonas, C. A., & Rosenblum, G. D. (1993). Assessment of binge eating in obese patients. *International Journal of Eating Disorders, 13*, 25–33.

Wing, R. R. (1998). Behavioral approaches to the treatment of obesity. In G. Bray, C. Bouchard, & P. T. James (Eds.), *Handbook of obesity* (pp. 855–873). New York: Marcel Dekker.

Wiser, S., & Telch, C. F. (1999). Dialectical behavior therapy for binge-eating disorder. *Journal of Clinical Psychology, 55*, 755–768.

Wisniewski, L., & Kelly, E. (2003). The application of dialectical behavior therapy to the treatment of eating disorders. *Cognitive and Behavioral Practice, 10*, 131–138.

Wisniewski, L., Safer, D., & Chen, E. Y. (2007). Dialectical behavior therapy and eating disorders. In L. A. Dimeff & K. Koerner (Eds.), *Dialectical behavior therapy in clinical practice: Applications across disorders and settings*. New York: Guilford Press.

Yanovski, S. Z., Nelson, J. E., Dubbert, B. K., & Spitzer, R. L. (1993). Association of binge eating disorder and psychiatric comorbidity in obese subjects. *American Journal of Psychiatry, 150*(10), 1472–1479.

Index

"a" indicates an appendix; *"f"* indicates a figure; *"n"* indicates a footnote; *"t"* indicates a table.

Absences from sessions. *See* Missed sessions
Abstinence. *See* Commitment to abstinence;
    Dialectical abstinence
Abstinence rates, 14–15
Acceptance and change balance, strategies,
    22–23
Accepting Reality skills, 155–169
    Awareness Exercises in, 161–162
    Burning Your Bridges in, 167–168, 178*a*
    case illustration, 201–202
    versus Crisis Survival skills, 155–156
    function of, 155–156
    Half-Smiling exercise, 159–161
    illustrative example, 156–157
    "Observing Your Breath" in, 157–159
    and Radical Acceptance, 162–167
    review of, 184
Acting Opposite to the Current Emotion skill,
    141–146
    bingeing/purging replacement, 145
    experiential exercise, 145–146
    homework practice, 146
    repetition as key, 142–143
    review of, 183
Adaptive skills. *See* Skills training
Adolescent clients, modifications, 215–218
Adult Pleasant Events Schedule, 138, 154*a*
    adolescent modifications, 217
Affect regulation. *See also* Emotion
    dysregulation model
    in binge-eating disorder, 8–9
    in bulimia nervosa, 12–13
Aftereffects of emotions, identification, 124,
    149*a*

Alcohol abuse. *See* Substance abuse/
    dependence
Alternate Rebellion Homework Sheet, 119*a*
Alternate Rebellion skill, 110–111, 119*a*
    case illustrations, 198–199, 211
    in Mindfulness module, 110–111, 119*a*,
    182
Anger, Acting Opposite skill, 144–145
Anxiety, anxiety disorders, 3*t*, 9–10
    Acting Opposite skill with, 141–143
Apparently irrelevant behaviors (AIBs)
    as treatment target, 37, 54–55, 82*a*, 85*a*
Assessments, in DBT for BED/BN research
    studies, 223–224
Avoid Avoiding skill, 140, 153*a*
Avoidant personality disorder, 10
Awareness exercises, purpose of, 161–162
Axis I diagnosis, comorbid, 3, 3*t*, 7, 10
Axis II disorders, comorbid, 3, 3*t*, 7, 10

B

Bariatric surgery, 7
Behavioral chain analysis
    case illustration, 196
    in depth review with client, 61–65
    guidelines for filling out, 57, 78*a*
    introduction to, 57–59
    problem behavior identification in, 57–58
    sample of, 57, 75*a*–77*a*
    sample of (blank copy), 79*a*–81*a*
    troubleshooting, 63–65
Behavioral weight-loss therapy, 13

Binge-eating disorder (BED)
  dialectical behavior therapy rationale, 5–15
  distinguishing characteristics, 5–6
  emotion and affect regulation, 8–9, 18–19
  gender ratio, 6
  physiological consequences, 8
  social/occupational impairment, 7–8
Bingeing (and purging). *See also* Binge-eating
      disorder; Bulimia nervosa
  biosocial model, 18–20, 50–52
  case illustration, group format, 203–213
  case illustration, individual format, 190–203
  chain analysis, 57–59
  and commitment to abstinence, 43–48,
      65–67, 88a
  dialectical abstinence approach, 20–21,
      65–67, 88a
  in emotion regulation model, 13, 18–19,
      33–34, 36, 48–49, 53–55
  as emotional "quick fix," 134–135
  mindfulness incompatibility, 92–94
Biosocial model, binge eating (and purging),
      18–20, 50–52
Body mass index, binge-eating disorder, 8
"Booster" group sessions, 218–219
Borderline personality disorder
  and binge-eating disorder, 7
  and bulimia nervosa, 10
  dialectical behavior therapy effectiveness,
      3–4, 17–18
Breathing exercises, 157–159
Building mastery activities, 137, 139f, 153a
Bulimia nervosa (BN). *See also* Bingeing (and
      purging)
  case illustration, 190–214
  diagnosis, 9
  dialectical behavior therapy rationale, 13–14
  emotions and affect regulation, 12–13, 18–
      19
  onset and course, 10
  physiological consequences, 11–12
  prevalence and symptomatology, 10–11
Burning Your Bridges homework sheet, 178a
Burning Your Bridges skill, 167–169
  case illustration, 202
  experiential exercise, 167–168
  homework practice, 169, 178a

C

Capitulation, as treatment target, 37, 54
Case examples
  group format, binge-eating disorder, 204–
      213
  individual format, bulimia nervosa, 190–203

CD-ROM support, 219
Chain analysis
  case illustrations, 196–197, 208–209
  dysfunctional links identification, 61, 87a
  and egregious-behavior protocol, 58n
  in group homework review, 26–29
  guidelines for filling out, 57, 78a
  in-depth review with client, 61–65
  introduction to, 57–59
  problem behavior identification, 57–58
  sample of, 57, 75a–77a, 79a–81a
  in skills practice report, 60–61
  troubleshooting, 63–65
Chain-analysis monitoring form, 23, 75a–77a,
      79a–81a
Chinese "finger puzzle," 129
Cognitive-behavioral therapy
  abstinence rates, DBT comparison, 15
  versus DBT, rationale, 13
Commitment to abstinence from bingeing (and
      purging)
  case illustration, group format, 206
  case illustration, individual format, 193–196
  dialectical abstinence in, 20–21, 65–67, 88
  eliciting and obtaining verbal commitment,
      43–44, 45–47
  homework practice, 47–48, 67
  maintenance of, future directions, 218–219
  renewing commitment, 179–180
  therapist techniques, 24–25, 43–48
Commitment, motivational strategies, 24–25,
      43–44, 46–47
Commitment to treatment, pretreatment
      interview, 32
Communication, emotions function, 130–133
Comorbid psychopathology
  in DBT for binge-eating disorder study, 3, 3t
  as treatment contraindication, 3–4
Confidentiality, 56
Connecting Present Commitments to Prior
      Commitments, 25
Contraindications to Adapted DBT treatment,
      3–4
"Conveyer belt" exercise, 101
Coping Ahead skill, 184–185
Cost-effectiveness of DBT adapted for BED/BN,
      improving, 221–222
Counting Your Breaths skill, 158–159
Cravings
  as treatment target, 37, 54
  Urge Surfing skill in, 108–110, 118a
Crisis Survival skills, 169–176
  case illustration, 201–202
  Distraction skills, 170–171
  experiential exercise, 173–174
  function, 155, 169

homework practice, 176
Improving the Moment in, 172–173
overview, 170
review of, 184
Self-Soothing in, 171–172
Thinking of Pros and Cons in, 174–175
troubleshooting, 175
Current emotion
Acting Opposite to skill, 141–146
Mindfulness of, 126–130

D

Deep breathing. *See* Diaphragmatic breathing
Dental complications, bulimia nervosa, 11
Depression
and Acting Opposite skill, 144
and binge-eating disorder, 7, 9
and bulimia nervosa, 10, 12
"Describe" skill
experiential exercise, 101
homework sheet, 116*a*
in Mindfulness, 100–101
in Mindfulness of Your Current Emotion, 126–128
review of, 182
troubleshooting, 102
Diabetes, 8, 12
Dialectical abstinence
in case illustration, group format, 209–210
in case illustration, individual format, 197
essence of, 20–21, 65–67
homework sheet, instructions for practicing, 88*a*
in introductory sessions protocol, 65–67
Olympic athlete metaphor, 66–67, 209
versus "touchdown every time" concept, 65*n*
Dialectical behavior therapy (DBT)
affect regulation model, 13–14
empirical evidence for, DBT adapted for BED/BN, 14–15
empirical evidence for, standard DBT, 17–18
philosophical influences, 17
Dialectical behavior therapy for BED/BN
adolescent clients, 215–218
Distress Tolerance module, 155–178
Emotion Regulation module, 120–154
future directions, 215–222
group sessions structure, 26–29
Mindfulness module, 89–119
pretreatment stage, 30–68
rationale for development of, 13–14, 16–21
research evidence, 14–15
therapist strategies, 22–25
weight loss adaptation of, 220–221

Dialectical philosophy, 17
Dialectical strategies, in treatment delivery, 22–25
Diaphragmatic breathing, 67–69
Diary cards
in group homework review, 26–29
homework practice, 59
instructions for filling out, 84*a*–85*a*
introduction to, 59
sample (blank copy) of, 82*a*–83*a*
troubleshooting, 64
Dieting, treating policy rationale, 21, 40–41
Distraction skills, 170–171
Distress Tolerance module, 155–178
Accepting Reality in, 155–169
adolescent clients, 216
case illustrations, 201–202, 212–213
client orientation, 39, 55
Crisis Survival skills, 169–176
function, 155–156
list of skills in, 177*a*
review of, 184
session by session content, 226–227
Door-in-the-Face techniques, 25
Drug abuse. *See* Substance abuse/dependence
Dysfunctional links, in chain analysis, 61, 87*a*

E

Effect sizes, DBT treatment, 15
"Effectively" skill, 107–108
homework sheet, 117*a*
in Mindfulness, 107–108
review of, 182
"Emotion diary," 135
Emotion dysregulation model, 70*a*. *See also* Affect regulation
and dialectical behavior therapy, 13–14, 18–19
explanation to client, 33–34, 70*a*, 191–193
and invalidating environments, 19–20
in orientation to treatment, 48–52
rationale of, 18–21
treatment effect size evidence, 15
Emotion Dysregulation Model of Problem Eating, 70*a*
Emotion Mind
bingeing (and purging) influence, 95, 97
definition, 95
homework practice, 98, 114*a*
reducing vulnerability to, 136–138, 139*f*, 153*a*, 200–201
Emotion Mind Homework Sheet, 114*a*
Emotion Regulation Model. *See* Emotion Dysregulation Model of Problem Eating

Emotion Regulation module, 120–154
  adolescent clients, 217
  case illustration, group format, 211–212
  case illustration, individual format, 199–201
  describing emotions model in, 121–126,
      149a
  function of emotions in, 130–133, 152a
  Mindfulness of current emotion in, 126–130
  positive emotions in, 138, 140–141
  pretreatment orientation, 38, 54–55
  primary and secondary emotions in, 124–
      125, 150a
  reducing vulnerability to Emotion Mind,
      136–138, 139f, 153a, 200–201
  review of, 183
  session by session content, 225–226
  versus skillful emotion regulation behaviors,
      more broadly defined, 38n2
  skills training goals, 20–21
  Wise Mind approach, 132–133
Emotional Eating Scale, 14–15, 224
Emotional sensitivity, bingeing (and purging)
      link, 50
Emotions. See also Current emotion
  function of, 130–135, 152a
  justified versus unjustified, 133–135
  model for describing of, 121–126, 149a, 161
  myths about, 146–147
  primary versus secondary, 124–125, 150a
  quotes about, 214
Empathy, balance with irreverence, therapist
      stylistic strategy, 24
Evaluating Pros and Cons strategy
  case illustration, 205–206
  in commitment to abstinence, 43–44, 47–48
  therapist role, 25
Exclusion criteria, 223
Exercise, emotional vulnerability reduction,
      137
Extending strategy, therapist role, 23

F

Facial expressions, physiology, 161
Family sessions, adolescents, 218
Fear, Acting Opposite skill, 143
Feedback session, 187
Final session, 187
"Finger puzzle" lesson, 129
Food preoccupation. See Preoccupation with
      food
Foot-in-the-Door techniques, 25, 46
Function of Emotions. See Emotions
Future directions, 215–222

G

Gender ratio
  binge-eating disorder, 6
  bulimia nervosa, 10
Glycemic control, binge-eating disorder, 8
Goals of Treatment, Goals of Skills Training,
      and Treatment Targets
  handout, 71a
  introductory sessions approach, 53–55
  orienting the client to, as part of
      pretreatment interview, 34–35
Group Member Treatment Agreements
  copy of, 72a
  in introductory sessions, 56–57
  in pretreatment interview, 31, 42
Group sessions
  homework review, 26–28, 86a
  orientation, 55–56
  skills instruction, 28–29
  structure, 26–29, 55–56
Guidelines for Filling Out a Behavioral Chain
      Analysis of a Problem Behavior, 78a
Guilt, 143–144

H

Half-smiling skill, 159–161
  experiential exercise, 160
  homework practice, 161
  physiology, 161
Health status, binge-eating disorder, 8
Highlighting Freedom to Choose in the
      Absence of Alternatives, 25, 47
Homework
  case illustration, group format, 206–210
  case illustration, individual format, 196–197
  commitment to binge (and purge) abstinence,
      47–48
  review in group sessions, 26–28, 86a
  troubleshooting, 63–65
"How Skills." See Mindfulness "How" skills
Hypnosis, mindfulness differences, 92
Hypokalemia, bulimia nervosa, 11–12

I

Imaginal mindful eating, 107
Improving the Moment skill, 172–173
Inclusion and exclusion criteria, 223
Individual Client Treatment Agreements
  copy of, 73a
  in pretreatment interview, 31, 42

Individual therapy, group skills combination, 60
Instructions for filling out a diary card, 84a–85a
Interpersonal effectiveness skills, 2, 38n3
  adolescents, 217
Interpersonal psychotherapy
  abstinence rates, DBT comparison, 15
  versus DBT, rationale, 13
Interpretations, emotional experiencing role, 122
Introductory sessions, 42–69
  adolescent clients, 216
  case illustrations, group format, 204–210
  case illustrations, individual format, 193–197
  chain analysis introduction, 57–63
  commitment to abstinence, 43–48
  and dialectical abstinence, 65–66
  diary card introduction, 59
  orientation to treatment, 48–55
  session by session content, 224
  treatment agreements in, 56–57
Invalidating environments
  consequences, 19–20, 50–52
  illustration of, 51–52
  therapeutic approach, 52
Irreverence. See Stylistic strategies

J

Judgmental thinking. See "Nonjudgmental" skill
Justified versus unjustified emotions, 133–135

L

Lateness to sessions, 40
Laxative use, 12
List of Distress Tolerance Skills, 177a
List of Emotion Regulation Skills, 148a
List of Mindfulness Core Skills, 112a
Loving Your Emotions skill, 128–130

M

Making Lemonade Out of Lemons strategy, 23
Malt balls, in Urge Surfing exercise, 109, 197–198
Matching clients, preliminary recommendation, 3
Meditation, mindfulness differences, 92

Men, binge-eating disorder, 6
"Mental Stimulation," 184n. See also Coping Ahead skill
Mindful eating. See also Mindfulness module; Path to Mindful Eating
  experiential exercises, 103, 107
  homework practice, 104, 116a
  imaginal exercises, 107
  path to, 71a, 221f
  review of, 182
  troubleshooting, 104
  in weight-loss oriented adaptation, 220
  "What" skills, 102, 103
Mindfulness "How" skills
  homework sheet, 117a
  orientation to, 104–108
  review of, 181–182
  troubleshooting, 108
Mindfulness "How" Skills Homework Sheet, 117
Mindfulness module, 89–119
  adolescent clients, 216–217
  alternate rebellion, 110–111, 119a
  and Awareness Exercises, 162
  binge-eating (and purging) incompatibility, 92–94, 98
  case illustration, group format, 210–211
  case illustration, individual format, 197–199
  core skills, 89–119
    list of, 112a
  and current emotion, 126–128
  definitions, 90–92
  function of, 38, 54
  "How" skills, 104–108, 117a
  meditation differences, 92
  mindful eating, 102–104
  session by session content, 225
  states of mind influence, 94–98
  troubleshooting difficulties, 91–92
  urge surfing, 108–110, 118a
  "What" skills, 99–102, 116a
Mindfulness of Your Current Emotion skill, 126–128
Mindfulness "What" skills
  homework, 104, 116a
  orientation to, 99–101
  review of, 181–182
  troubleshooting difficulties, 102
Mindfulness "What" Skills Homework Sheet, 104, 116a
Mindless eating
  treatment target, orienting the client to, 36–37, 71a
  treatment target, therapist review of, 53, 71a

Missed sessions
   group member agreements, 56–57
   pretreatment interview orientation, 32, 32n
Model for Describing Emotions, 121–126, 149a
Mood states
   binge-eating disorder, 7, 8–9
   bulimia nervosa, 10–11, 12–13
   emotional states distinction, 121
Mortality rate, bulimia nervosa, 11
Motivation
   commitment to abstinence link, 43–48
   function of emotions link, 131–132
   therapist role, 24–25

N

Naming an emotion, 123–124, 149a
Negative emotion/mood
   binge-eating disorder, 8–9
   bulimia nervosa, 12–13
   emotional vulnerability link, 19
"Nonjudgmental" skill, 104–106
   homework sheet, 117a
   overview, 104–106
   review of, 182

O

Obesity
   binge-eating overlap, 6–8
   correlation with binge-eating severity, 8
   as treatment target, 220–221
"Observe" skill, 99–100
   experiential exercises, 99, 101
   homework sheet, 116a
   in identifying an emotion's trigger, model for
     emotions, 121–122
   in Mindfulness of Your Current Emotion,
     126–128
   review of, 182
Observing and Describing Emotions, 126–127
   homework sheet, 127f, 152a
Observing Your Breath skill, 157–158
   and Coping Ahead, 185
   experiential exercise, 157–158
   homework practice, 159
   review of, 184
Occupational impairment, 7–8, 11
Olympic athlete metaphor, 66–67, 209
"One-Mindfully" skill, 106–107
   experiential exercise, 107
   homework sheet, 117a
   review of, 182

Online support, 219
Outcome of treatment, case example, 203
Outpatients, 2
Overweight
   versus binge eating, loss of control, 93–94
   as treatment target, 220–221

P

"Participate" skill, 101
   homework sheet, 116a
Path to Mindful Eating, 71a, 221f
   orienting client to, 35–39
Personality disorders, 3t, 7, 10
Planning for the Future, 186–187
   case illustration, group format, 213
   case illustration, individual format, 202–203
   goal of, 186
   homework practice, 186–187, 189a
Planning for the Future Homework Sheet,
   189a
Playing the Devil's Advocate, 25, 44
Positive experiences/emotions
   Adult Pleasant Events schedule, 154a
   homework practice, 139f, 141, 153a
   increasing Mindfulness of, 140–141
   steps for increasing of, 138, 140–141
Preoccupation with food
   treatment target, introductory sessions
     review, 54, 71a
   treatment target, pretreatment interview
     orientation, 37, 71a
   Urge Surfing skill in, 108–110, 118a
Pretreatment interview, 31–42
   case illustration, group format, 204
   case illustration, individual format, 191–193
   emotion dysregulation model in, 33–34
   general treatment issues, 39–42
   goals, 31–32
   mindful eating path orientation, 35–39
Pretreatment stage, 30–69
   content, 224
   introductory sessions as part of, 42–69
   pretreatment interview as part of, 31–42
Primary emotions
   and emotion regulation, 124–125, 150
   homework sheet, 150a
   versus secondary emotions, 124–125
Primary Emotions and Secondary Reactions
   Homework Sheet, 150a
Problem behavior
   in chain analysis, 57–59, 61–63, 75a, 78a,
     79a
   in skills practice report, 60–61, 86a

Problem solving, therapist strategies, 23–24
Prompting events
    bingeing and purging, 48–49
    in chain analysis, 58, 62–63, 75a, 78a, 79a
    in describing emotions model, 121–124,
        149
Pros and Cons strategy. *See* Evaluating Pros
    and Cons strategy

Q

Quality of life, impact of BED and BN, 8, 11
Quotes about Emotions, 214a

R

Radical Acceptance, 162–167
    case illustration, group format, 212–213
    case illustration, individual format, 201
    experiential exercises, 163–165
    versus passivity, 163–164
    review, 184
    troubleshooting, 166–167
    and Turning the Mind, 165
    Willingness and Willfulness in, 165–166
Randomized controlled trials of DBT adapted
        for BED/BN, 14–15
Reasonable Mind
    definition, 94–95
    homework practice, 98, 115a
    review of, 181
Reasonable Mind Homework Sheet, 115a
Recommitting to stop bingeing (and purging),
        168
Reducing Vulnerability to Emotion Mind. *See*
        Emotion Regulation module
Relapse, 10, 218
Relapse prevention, 184–189, 218–219
Remission, bulimia nervosa, 10
Research evidence, DBT adaptation for BED
        and BN, 14–15
Review of skills, 181–184

S

Sadness, Acting Opposite skill, 144
Sample Chains Focusing on Key Dysfunctional
        Link(s), 87a
Secondary emotions
    and emotion regulation, 124–125, 150a
    homework sheet, 150a
    versus primary emotions, 124–125

Self-injury
    affect regulation model, 13
    standard dialectical behavioral therapy
        effectiveness, 17–18
Self-invalidation, consequences, 19–20
Self-Soothing skill, 171–172, 202
Self-validation. *See* Validation
Sensitivity. *See* Emotional sensitivity
Shame, 143–144
Skills practice
    in group homework review, 26–29
    guidelines, 86a
    structuring client's report of, 60–61, 86a
    troubleshooting, 63–65
Skills training
    goals, 20–22, 71a
    in group sessions, 28–29
    in individual therapy, 60
    orientation of client to, 34–35, 38–39
Sleep, decreasing emotional vulnerability link,
        137
Social impairment
    binge-eating disorder, 7–8
    bulimia nervosa, 11
Solution-analysis strategy, 23–24
Steps for Reducing Painful Emotions
        Homework Sheet, 138, 139f, 153a
Structural treatment strategies, 25
Structure of sessions, 22–29
    orientation to, 55–56
Structuring Client's Report of Skills Practice,
        60–61, 63–65, 86a
Stylistic strategies, 24
Substance abuse/dependence
    and binge-eating disorder, 3, 3t, 7
    and bulimia nervosa, 3, 10
    and DBT effectiveness, 18
    treatment contraindication, 3–4
Suffering, as nonacceptance of pain, 164
Suicidality, 3, 17–18
    contraindication for adapted DBT, 3–4
Synopsis of Ways to Describe Emotions,
        125–126, 151a

T

Team consultations, strategies, 25
Termination of treatment, 180–181
Therapist Treatment Agreements, 74a
    in introductory sessions, 56–57
    in pretreatment interview, 31, 42
Therapists
    essential "attitude" of, 22–23
    in group sessions homework review, 26–28

Therapists *(cont.)*
  skills instruction/training, 20–21, 28–29
  stylistic aspects, 24
  in treatment delivery, 22–25
Therapy-interfering behavior
  case illustration, group format, 206–210
  case illustration, individual format, 196–197
  intervention top priority, 36–37
  review of, 53
Thinking of Pros and Cons skill, 174–175
Treatment goals
  introductory sessions review, 53–55
  orientation of client to, 34–35
Treatment model, assumptions, rationale, 48–49.
    See also Emotion Dysregulation Model of
    Problem Eating
Treatment protocol, adherence, 21
Treatment team, consultation strategies, 25
Treatment termination, 180–181
Turning the Mind, 165

U

Ugly duckling story, 129
Urge Surfing Homework sheet, 118*a*
Urge Surging skill, 108–110
  case illustration, group format, 210–211
  case illustration, individual format, 197–198
  experiential exercise, 109
  homework sheet, 118*a*
  review of, 182
  troubleshooting, 109
Urges, as treatment target, 37, 54

V

Validation, 22–23, 52, 133
Verbal commitment to abstinence, 45–47
Vulnerability factors, in chain analysis, 58

W

"Ways to Describe Emotions," 125–126,
    151*a*
Weight, weight loss
  abstinence from bingeing benefit, 220
  policy explanation to client, 40–41
  targeting, 220–221
  as treatment secondary priority, 21, 40–
    41
Weight preoccupation, 7
"What" skills. *See* Mindfulness "What" skills
Willingness and Willfulness, 165–166
Wise Mind
  definition, 95
  in emotion validation, 132–133
  experiential exercise, 97
  homework practice, 98, 113*a*
  "How" skills access to, 104–108
  practice in accessing of, 97
  review of, 181
  therapist's self-disclosure example, 96
  "What" skills access to, 99–102
Wise Mind Homework Sheet, 113*a*
Women
  binge-eating disorder prevalence, 6
  bulimia nervosa prevalence, 10